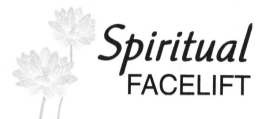

# *Spiritual*
## FACELIFT

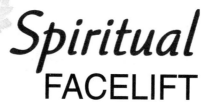

# *Spiritual* FACELIFT

### 7 Natural Steps to Inner and Outer Health and Beauty

# Victoria Holt

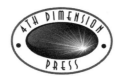

4th Dimension Press ■ Virginia Beach ■ Virginia

4th Dimension Press
215 67th Street
Virginia Beach, VA 23451-2061


ISBN-13: 978-0-87604-625-8 (trade paper)

All scripture quotations in this book were taken from THE HOLY BIBLE,
NEW INTERNATIONAL VERSION®, NIV®. Copyright © 1973, 1978, 1984 by
Biblica US, Inc.®.

**Disclaimer**
The contents of this publication are intended for educational and infor-
mative use only. They are not to be considered directive nor as a guide
to self-diagnosis or self-treatment. Before embarking on any therapeu-
tic regimen, it is absolutely essential that you consult with and obtain
the approval of your personal physician or health care provider.

Cover design by Christine Fulcher

This book is dedicated to
every person who has not yet discovered
that true beauty comes from the heart.
May you learn to love yourself unconditionally
and remember that you are a unique and perfect child of God.

# Contents

# Acknowledgments

I have so many people to thank. Without your love and support this book would not have been published. I have so much gratitude for each and every one of you that I felt you had to have an individual acknowledgment. Thank you all—I love you so very much and deeply appreciate all that you have done for me.

**Cassie McQuagge** and **4th Dimension Press**—Thank you for believing in this book. You are an amazing team to work with. Let us make this a bestseller!

**Stephanie Pope**—Thank you! You are an amazingly supportive and brilliant editor!

**Josie Varga**—Thank you for helping me secure a book deal. I am so very grateful.

**Stephen King** and **JK Rowling**—Thank you for your support and belief in my work. I could not have written this book without you.

**James Padgett**—The Divine Laws shared in Chapter 2 and the descriptions of God in Chapter 6 were originally recorded from 1914–1920 by James Padgett. Excerpts were taken from *The Book of Truths* and *Angelic Revelations of Divine Truth—Volumes 1 and 2*. Thank you, James, for all your hard work.

**AJ Miller**—Thank you for your intricate explanation and update of the Padgett Messages. Thank you also for your new revelations, many of which have been included in this book.

**Philip Permutt**—All the crystal prescriptions throughout the book are taken from the book *The Crystal Healer* by Philip Permutt.

**John Doel**—Thank you for creating the graphics in the book. I am eternally grateful.

**Jerid O'Connell**—Thank you for your quality work on the front cover.

**Neal Tabachnick**—Thank you for encouraging me to write *Spiritual Facelift*.

**Catriona Drummond**—Thank you for your help, belief, and support. You are the best!

**John Heatly**—I want to thank you for all your unconditional love and support for the last sixteen years. I am eternally grateful to you for your belief in me. God sent me an angel when I met you. You are one of the kindest souls on the planet. I love you, my dear friend.

**Diana Heatly**—Thank you for your love and support. You, too, are an angel.

**Gilly**—Thank you for helping me throughout five difficult years in seclusion and for believing in my spiritual journey. I love you, and I'm deeply grateful.

**Ken**—Thank you for your love and support, especially during the dark days.

**Anne, Lizzie,** and **Nicky Holt**—Thank you for being such a caring and loving family.

**Amy Platt**—Thank you for being the most wonderful niece. You embody true beauty.

**Mae Chee Sansanee** and **Joy**—Thank you for believing in my work and loving me.

**Mother Maya**—Thank you for your loving guidance while I was walking "through the fire."

**Michael Head**—Thank you for twenty years of brotherly friendship, love, and laughter.

**Justin Southgate**—Thank you for your never-ending support and belief in me.

**Liane Weintraub** and **Victoria Wachtel**—Thank you, beautiful ladies, for supporting my work.

**Jacqueline Beaudette**—Thank you, soul sister, for sharing the Ascension journey.

**Charlie** and **Karen Vitale**—Thank you for believing in me and supporting my work.

**Barbara Zaneri**—Thank you for cheering on my book.

**Rushick** and **LeGrande**—Thank you for believing in me so strongly and working with me.

**Rita Safady**—Thanks for your friendship and helping me through my period of seclusion.

**Robert Johnson**—Thank you for your loving kindness and chiropractic back support!

**Lottie Ross**—Thank you for thirty years of sisterly friendship and a lifetime of love.

**Keith Bryan** and **The Old Blues Society**—Thank you for your kind support.

**Mika Sogawa**—Thank you for sharing the journey.

**Michael Kane**—Thank you for helping me through the worst time of my life!

**Gabriella Orlando**—Thank you, my Italian sister, for sharing the journey.

**Tina Nail** and **Michael Rockett**—Thank you for years of friendship, love, and support.

**Susan Young-Kravitz**—Thanks for securing the perfect winter nest to write this book.

**Beau** and **Hero**—Thank you for being my constant, loving furry companions.

Finally, I want to thank God and my spirit guides for the guidance and help I have received throughout my lifetime. I also want to thank my father and other deceased family members and spirits who help me from the Other Side. I want to also send love to my soul mate. May you one day awaken to Divine Truth and find your way home to me and to God.

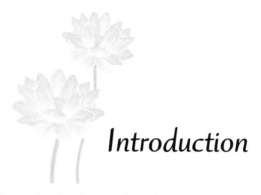

# Introduction

*The recipe for beauty is to have less illusion and more soul . . .*
**Mary Baker Eddy**

Welcome to *Spiritual Facelift*. Thank you for joining me on this exciting journey of rejuvenation. I am delighted to share with you this revolutionary self–help book on natural health and beauty that says, "Put down that knife and get on with your life!" I believe your soul has guided you to read this book. You are not just ready to renew your body but to change your life and elevate your level of spiritual understanding.

Every year billions of dollars are spent on the health and beauty industry as many strive to keep themselves looking young and beautiful. The desire for youthful beauty has become such an obsession that many feel compelled to inject their faces with poison or go under the knife to have their body parts cut away. These unnatural procedures and cosmetic surgeries not only cost a fortune but also damage bodies and endanger lives. This endless search for eternal youth and physical perfection is creating low self-esteem and depression, not to mention an empty wallet whose content has paid for a plastic surgeon's million-dollar home but failed to buy any long–term happiness.

I was inspired to write *Spiritual Facelift* so that both women and men learn to stop harming themselves and discover the real meaning of true beauty. I want to free us all from the myth of perfection. *Spiritual Facelift* is a guide to both inner and outer natural health and beauty. In these hard economic times, it is THE cost–effective, safe, and painless choice to stop the aging process. It teaches you how to tap into the eternal fountain of youth the natural way.

This book is packed full of powerful ancient and modern–day spiritual wisdoms, natural remedies, and practical tips that will change deeply the cellular makeup of everyone who reads it. No matter your age, faith, ethnicity, or gender, this spiritual health and beauty program will transform your appearance and your life.

I have been teaching spirituality to both individuals and global audiences for many years. Throughout my journey, I have spent intimate time working with some of the world's most revered spiritual leaders. I noticed that they were different from other people I had met. They were able to work twenty hours a day without getting tired; they looked very young for their age and had amazing skin. Despite wearing simple robes and no makeup, they had a beauty that went far beyond that of any supermodel I had seen gracing the covers of the world's top magazines.

Then I began to notice that the more I followed my own spiritual practice, the more my appearance changed. People were commenting that I was looking younger and more radiant every time they saw me. After a bout of serious illness, a painful divorce, and a job loss, I felt guided to go deeper into my own spiritual practice and change my life. For the next five years I lived in near seclusion studying many ancient spiritual texts and absorbing teachings from an array of diverse spiritual disciplines. I wanted to find a connecting thread of Divine Truth amongst the different paths. I began to purify my mind, my body, and my soul—learning to become a spiritual master (who wears designer clothes instead of a robe!) The more my soul purified, the more spiritual truth was given to me. These revelations led me to the secret of how to tap into the fountain of eternal youth. I want to share these secrets with you in *Spiritual Facelift*.

*Spiritual Facelift* is non–denominational. It contains an array of teachings that you can apply to your current spiritual practice or religious belief system. Through my own process of spiritual purification, my soul experienced a fundamental shift of consciousness as I received vast amounts of divine information. This sacred knowledge has since been corroborated by other spiritual teachers and individuals who have been through the same deep soul training. I also discovered the same spiritual information in sacred books called *The Book of Truths* and the *Angelic Revelations of Divine Truth—Volumes 1 and 2*. The information in the books was recorded by James Padgett from 1914–1920. I received further revelations from spiritual teacher AJ Miller who shared updated information on the Padgett messages. Both sources also confirmed all of my own personal spiritual experiences and conclusions.

The teachings in *Spiritual Facelift* took me many years to learn, but if you follow the spiritual and practical paths in this book, you can start getting results and changing your looks and your life in just a few weeks. I encourage you to travel on the same journey and not just intellectually accept the truths presented in this book. I approached all of my spirit training in the manner of an investigative journalist. There is nothing written in this book that I have not personally experienced as Divine Truth. Many of the teachings are new, and some may feel challenging at first. Aligning your life with God's Truth can sometimes feel uncomfortable because it challenges us to overcome fears and release emotional injuries as well as ingrained belief systems that are not harmonious with love. I encourage you to question but to also stay open to the new information in this book so that your soul not only opens to Divine Truth but actually experiences it as I did.

By reading *Spiritual Facelift* and following the seven steps with their array of exciting exercises, you will no longer feel the need to put your body and life at risk. You will realize that staying young and beautiful, the natural way, is the only way to live. The book will guide you to the root cause of why you are aging and creating wrinkles along with excess body fat. Your body will go through a metamorphosis as it becomes more youthful and radiant; all without having to spend a single dollar on dermatologists or plastic surgery. You will not only save money but most importantly you will also keep yourself safe from poisons and sharp knives. By following the practices in *Spiritual Facelift*, you will discover that there is no need for diet pills, liposuction, facelifts,

Botox, tummy tucks, breast implants, or dangerously invasive fat-sucking machines. You can become your own spiritual master, healer, dermatologist, and fitness trainer as you reshape and rejuvenate your body from the safety and comfort of your home.

I believe this book will not only change your appearance but will also change your life. *Spiritual Facelift* is an A–Z guide to living. Your whole life will be given a top-to-toe makeover as you gain a deeper understanding of who you are and why you are alive. As you change your relationship to your mind, body, and soul, you will learn how to change your relationship with yourself and the world around you. *Spiritual Facelift* will help you create healthy relationships, manifest abundance, discover your soul purpose, and create a dream life.

All the chapters in the book are individually tailored to help each part of your body and all areas of your life reach their highest potential. At the beginning of each chapter you will be given all the spiritual information you need to understand the root cause of your aging, weight issues, and life problems while at the end of each chapter you will be given practical, mental, emotional, spiritual, and physical exercises to reverse physical damage and make over your life.

I hope you will share the contents of this book with friends, family, your partner, and even your children so that they, too, can learn to live to their highest potential and discover the real meaning of true beauty. Age and true beauty are not defined by a number or a dress size but by the contents of your soul. Live from your eternal soul and you will stay young and beautiful forever more.

Victoria Holt

# 1
# Why Do We Age?

*People do not grow old no matter how long we live.*
*We never cease to stand like curious children*
*before the Great Mystery into which we were born.*
**Albert Einstein**

Most people who love their lives want to tap into the fountain of youth and live longer. Each year men and women, especially, spend thousands of their hard-earned dollars, trying to extend their lives and recapture their youthful face and body. Some people give up their search for a wrinkle-free face; they accept their fate and try to grow old gracefully. They cannot afford the expense of new beauty gimmicks, and they would rather stay safe than die under a plastic surgeon's knife. But others are determined to continue waging a war against old age. They are consumed with their appearance and refuse to go down without a fight. In the process their looks become unnatural, and their lives become unbalanced. They dabble with dangerous life-threatening procedures and turn their God-given looks into something abnormal. They change into someone unrecognizable, wearing the same mass-produced face that the plastic surgeon has decided is the definition of beautiful.

So why, after all these centuries of inventions, potions, and sending men to the moon, have we not yet discovered how to tap naturally into that fountain of youth and stop ourselves from aging? Why are our

1

bodies still deteriorating and decaying?

This is the age-old question that has yet to be answered. But there are those who believe they have discovered how to reverse the aging process. These people are highly enlightened spiritual masters who say the secret of eternal youth does not come from a bottle or a quick-fix tummy tuck but through learning the real secret of life itself, thereby changing our perception about the body and fully awakening to who we are.

Spiritual masters look at their bodies in a totally different way from most other people. They see them simply as materialized energy whose purpose is to house and support the soul. They believe that both body and soul can return to a pure state of being and become eternal.

Many scientists are now joining forces with the spiritual community and beginning to back up these age-old spiritual theories. Ever since Einstein proved that $E=mc^2$, we have known that matter and energy are really different forms of the same thing. Matter is trapped energy. Now scientists are expanding Einstein's theories and confirming that everything in the universe is made up of energy—and that includes our physical body. They have concluded that our physical universe is not really composed of matter at all. Its basic component is a force or essence that we call energy, and this energy cannot die or be destroyed; it can only change form.

In the Hindu tradition energy is known as *prana*. It is believed to be the life-sustaining force which pervades all living organisms and the universe. The Chinese also believe that we are made up of energy—they call it Qi (pronounced Chi). Qi has been written about and studied for over ten thousand years from China and Japan to India, the Hawaiian Islands, and South America. The Chinese refer to Qi as the vital life force energy of the universe present within every living thing. It describes the relationship among matter, energy, and spirit. Chinese acupuncture is dedicated to ensuring the flow and balance of Qi through the body while Eastern martial art forms, such as Tai Chi or Qi Gong, base their practices on focusing and directing the flow of Qi.

It is important to know that you are not a solid physical being. You need to look at your body holistically with new eyes. When you look into the mirror, it gives out the appearance of something being solid, but in reality it is just pure energy. This may seem hard to grasp at first. As you touch your arm, it appears solid and made up of blood, bone, and tissue, but if you take a closer look, beyond your human everyday perception, you will discover that your body is not solid—it is, in fact, energy condensed into matter. If you still do not believe me, look through a microscope at the cells that make up your body; see how they break down into molecules and atoms. If you break down each atom further still, you will see that the atoms are made of ever smaller and smaller particles within particles. At their core these particles are made of pure energy.

## WHAT IS ENERGY?

You can actually feel your energy and the energy of other people. How often have people walked into a room and you have felt their energy before you know they are even there? People always say that someone has good energy or bad energy, and that is a true statement because the body is made up of nothing but energy. Once you accept and understand that everything is made up of energy, including you, then you will not only be able to tap into the fountain of youth but will finally answer the age-old question of life. But before you can start to reverse the aging process and learn how to tap into the fountain of youth, you need to understand what energy is and where it comes from.

What is this mysterious invisible substance called energy that fills your body and the whole universe and determines whether you die or live? Energy is the universal life force that connects all things. It is intelligent and is found in different forms, such as light, heat, sound, and motion. Energy has the ability to do work and change things. Energy moves cars along the street and propels airplanes across the sky. It makes a kettle boil or freezes water. It helps us watch our favorite television shows and powers lights. Energy allows our minds to think and our bodies to grow. Human beings are actually energy in motion.

So why then, if our bodies are made of an energy that can never expire or be destroyed, are we aging and dying? The answer lies in the frequency of our energy and the condition of our soul.

Energy moves in circular motion and creates a vibration or frequency.

This vibration can be perceived as a wave, and it stores information. The great scientist Nikola Tesla discovered that everything in nature has its own electromagnetic charge and resonant frequency. Everything in creation is made up of electromagnetic energy vibrating at different frequencies that correspond to sound, light, and color. He noted that these frequencies or energy vibrations, as they are also known, pulsate at a different rate and have different qualities. Frequencies can vary from fine, light qualities to dense, dark ones. When the energy is fine and light, it not only vibrates higher and faster but is also very quick and easy to change. When the vibration is dense, then it vibrates slowly and is sluggish. For example, rocks are dense and vibrate at a low frequency. They are, therefore, slower to change and more difficult to affect. We look at the pebbles on the shore and realize that they were once rocks worn down over the years by the action of the waves (another form of energy). In fact, all forms of energy such as earth, water, fire, and air are interconnected and affect one another.

Animals can register different vibrations more than humans can. They hear and transmit energy sound waves over long distances. Many natural disasters produce sound waves before the disaster manifests, and by observing the behavior of animals, humans can be forewarned of danger, especially in areas prone to earthquakes. For example, some people keep goldfish because a few hours before an earthquake the goldfish will begin to jump out of the bowl. During the Indonesian tsunami, elephants took to high ground before anyone knew that the water was coming. But even though the human ear is limited and cannot hear frequencies in the same way as animals, some people claim they can feel them. In fact, for some, this strong ability to sense frequencies can produce feelings of anxiety, sadness, headaches, nausea, and other kinds of mental, emotional, or physical disturbances.

Every part of your body—bones, muscle, organs, glands, etc.—has a specific frequency. The flesh of the human body is made of relatively fine, light energy; therefore, the body's frequency vibrates relatively fast and is very sensitive to change. It is affected by anything in or around it, including others people's energy, the external environment, natural elements, and the different substances that we ingest every day. Even our thoughts and emotions produce vibrations, which manifest as effects within our bodies and around us. The vibrations of our thoughts, beliefs, and emotions become embedded and carried in our DNA from generation to generation. When the flow of energy through the body is impeded by negatively charged emotions or destructive thought patterns, the cellular structure of our bodies becomes damaged. This results in disease and old age.

Close your eyes and feel the state of your energy. Are you full of energy or do you feel depleted and tired? Is your energy peaceful or angry and aggressive? Feel how your energy changes throughout the day. Now turn your attention to other people; see if you can feel their energy, too. When you say that people have good or bad energy, you are actually feeling the frequency of their energy field and the type of emotions in their soul. You are detecting whether they have a fine, light positive-energy vibration or a dense dark-energy field with a lower negative vibration. The same happens when you walk into a room; rooms absorb people's energy. You can feel if the energy is either positive and of a high vibration or dark and negative—a place you should run from.

Energy can also travel through time and space. You can learn to send an energy wave to someone deliberately. You can think of a friend, and the energies of your thoughts and feelings will make their way to him or her. Energy follows thoughts and emotions although many thoughts and emotions may be inaudible to our ears. When you focus on your friend, he or she will most probably call you within the next day or two and say, "I was thinking of you." Yes, of course that person was; you had sent out your energy. Energy can reach anyone, no matter how far away he or she lives.

You can actually fine-tune yourself to send and receive energy to such an extent that you will begin to feel someone sending you energy as well. Sometimes this energy is positive and helpful, but other times you may feel bad energy as well as negative feelings being sent to you even if that unfriendly person is living as far away as Australia!

When you learn to scan energy, there are no secrets; you will feel everything hidden underneath the surface. You will know if it is safe to have a person in your vicinity or whether or not you should stay away because his or her energy is dark and dangerous. The more you learn to read a person's energy, the more you will be kept safe in life, far from negative encounters and disruptive behaviors. You will learn to say "Yes," "No," "Thank you," "Hello," and "Goodbye" very quickly! This will save you time, keep unnecessary dramas at bay, and reduce your stress level.

## How You Have Damaged Your Physical Body

In the modern-day world, the energy of our bodies is constantly under attack from pollutants, toxic food, and life-style changes because of the stress we accumulate in our everyday lives. We use up too much of our energy, burn up our bodies, and put out our light. Our thoughts have become negative, and we hold onto painful emotions such as anger, shame, and fear that vibrate at a lower frequency than the energy of love. As we start to vibrate at a lower, slower frequency, our natural energy becomes dense and sluggish, and our bodies start to change. Our body struggles to release toxins, and our energy field becomes clogged. This weakens the body and affects its ability to heal quickly.

But our bodies are also being damaged not just by the junk food we eat or the negative emotions that contaminate our souls but because we have cut ourselves off from God's Divine Love and the universal life force that is meant to flow smoothly through our body at all times. Without this flow of pure loving energy, we cannot rejuvenate and replenish our cells, and we become far from being at one with God, a state of perfected love. We disconnect from the eternal fountain of youth. Pure energy feeds and nourishes us, and without it, our body and our energy field cannot get enough light. Without our natural light source, our body becomes dense, dark, contaminated, and depleted. It starts to fill up with the wrong kind of energy. This is the root cause of aging and why our cells and body die.

So how do you correct the damage that you have done to your body, reverse the aging process, and stay young, healthy, and vibrant without having to pay for plastic surgery and risk the permanent damage of an unnatural facelift, liposuction, or silicone implants? To start to self-heal and rejuvenate, you need to address the cause rather than treat the effect. Botox, facelifts, liposuction, or breast implants are short-term treatments for the effects. They do not address the cause of the long-term damage. If you can heal the cause, you can end your aging and body issue problems. But before you can start to do that, you first need to learn about the body's main energy system because it is here where blockages and the first stages of damage and aging occur.

Men and women spend much of their time focused on their physical body—grooming and pruning it, covering and adorning it. But if you want to stay truly young, healthy, and beautiful, you need to change your perception of your body further and understand that you do not have just one body, your physical body, to look after but you also have a *soul* and a *spirit body* (also known as the *etheric body* or *aura*) as well. It is your soul and your spirit body that determine the frequency of your energy and the state of your physical condition.

Your soul is an entity, the real you—your individuality and real self. Your individual soul is a container that stores all of your *passions, desires, emotions, aspirations, intentions, free will, memories, personality, instincts,* and *natural love.* The spirit body—the etheric layer—is the state between energy and matter or the border between the physical body and the soul. The spirit body and physical body (also known as the *material body*) are mere appendages of the soul. They exist because a soul cannot experience life without a body (either spirit body or a physical body.)

The seat of your soul—the foundation of the container—is your emotions; so much so that you can truthfully say that you are not only a soul but also an emotional being. Unfortunately, throughout history we have not been taught this. Mankind's focus has been on revering and perfecting the physical body and the intellectual mind instead of processing emotions and healing the soul—the real self.

The soul, the spirit body, and physical body are connected together by cords which allow energy and information to flow among the three parts. A gold cord connects the soul to the spirit body while a silver cord connects the spirit body to the physical body. The spirit body has a mind attached to it (the subconscious mind), and the physical body has a brain, which is the body's computer. The mind of the spirit body communicates with the brain, which, in turn, sends messages to the different body parts. But all thoughts and feelings are generated from the soul.

The condition of the soul is affected by *truth* or *error*—anything that enters and is retained by the soul that is harmonious with Divine Love is truthful or anything that enters and is retained by the soul that is disharmonious with Divine Love is an error. If your emotions and the contents of your soul are harmonious with love, then your energy stays pure and vibrates quickly which helps your body stay young. But unfortunately, more often than not, the contents of our souls are out of harmony with love and are thus negative and energetically dense. They cause us pain due to our error–based upbringing and societal belief systems. The soul expresses not only the happy but also the painful memories of childhood events which block the flow of energy and disrupt how the body functions. Damage starts to occur first in the soul, then in the spirit body, and finally in the physical body. The soul's condition and contents impact and are reflected in the spirit body which, in turn, impact the physical body.

When people "die," all that occurs is that their "real self" separates from the physical body. It is the breaking of the silver cord from the physical body that results in its death. Once the silver cord has snapped, the soul and the spirit body are no longer directly materially connected to the physical body. The physical body "dies" and the brain dissolves because they no longer receive a stream of life–force energy and information from the soul and the spirit body. The soul and spirit body always remain connected; they are never separated, even after death. They are now a "spirit" in that they have a soul and a spirit body but no material body. The person no longer resides in the physical (material) world but continues to exist in a nonphysical reality on the Other Side.

Let us discuss further your soul, your spirit body, and your physical body individually so that you have full understanding of the function and role of each. Once you understand the working systems of your soul, spirit body, and physical body, you will not only start to understand that everything is affected by your soul condition, but you will also understand what you are really looking at in the mirror.

Even though the soul, spirit body, and physical body are being discussed separately, remember that there are no impenetrable barriers between them; they coexist in the same space. If you continue to

## Diagram of the Soul, Spirit Body, and Physical Body

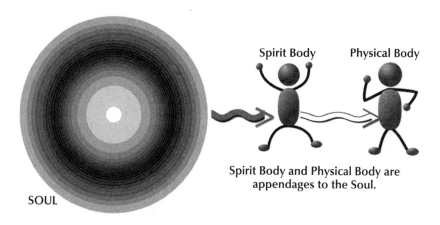

Spirit Body and Physical Body are
appendages to the Soul.

SOUL

At conception, our unaware soul is attracted in by our parents. It forms both a spirit body and physical body and starts the road of self-discovery. The spirit body is attached to the soul by a gold cord, and the physical body is attached to the spirit body by a silver cord through which a stream of life-force energy and information flows.

focus on only your physical body and ignore your soul and spirit body, you will be unhealthy and imbalanced. They are interdependent and need to work together optimally if your body is to stay young and healthy.

## THE SOUL

One secret to understanding God's universe is learning to understand the human soul. But to understand the soul and its workings fully we must first correct some of the myths about the soul. Your soul is an entity. It is the real you—the living, breathing, feeling, emotional, core of you. It is not your physical body nor as many New Age and Eastern gurus teach, is it your spirit body, etheric body, or aura. The spirit body and the physical body are mere appendages of the soul, created for each individual soul at conception.

All souls are created by God who is an infinite soul and entity—the Supreme Being. All souls are made in God's image; they are created by God's Desire and God's Sexual Union. The reason that souls incarnate and that you were born was so your soul could gain a consciousness of self and individualize. Before your soul incarnated, it was not conscious or self-aware. At conception your unaware soul was drawn in by your parents' Law of Attraction. Something in their souls attracted in your particular personality type. Your soul formed both a spirit body and physical body in your mother's womb and started the road of self-discovery.

Before your soul was born, it was part of a whole soul containing masculine as well as feminine qualities and energies. The whole soul is a reflection of God. God's infinite soul is also made up of masculine and feminine qualities and energies. When you were conceived, your whole soul split into two soul halves. These halves individualized and formed their own physical body and spirit body. It is these soul halves that are known as soul mates. You are one half of a soul-mate pair.

After separating from the whole soul, the two individualized soul halves continue on with their individual life experiences and soul journeys. Each half is complete in itself. The two halves do remain connected energetically at all times even if they never meet or live far apart. But throughout their lifetimes, each soul instinctively searches for the other and has a desire to reunite and become whole again although they are not consciously aware of this desire. As the two soul halves progress in love, they get drawn back together. They also continue to progress in love and evolve after they die. When they reach the highest level of love on the Other Side, the two halves release their individual spirit bodies and merge back together as one whole soul. At this point, reincarnation can happen. You will read more about soul mates and the soul split in Chapter 4.

There is much still to learn about the soul, such as the fact that it has a unique personality and holds many different attributes and qualities. Even though souls are created in the same way by God, each individual soul is completely different from another—each soul is unique. Your individual soul contains only your passions, desires, emotions, aspirations, intentions, free will, memories, personality, instincts, and natural love.

Your soul also has senses, which it uses to gather information and experience the universe. The soul picks up and retains emotional residue from others. Emotions from the soul become stored in both the spirit body and the cells of the physical body. If these emotions are loving, they positively impact the body. If they are disharmonious and negative, they cause physical damage.

Your individualized soul half was incarnated so that you could not only become self-aware but also experience your environment and your own free will. It also incarnated to develop a natural love for everything in that environment and to develop a personal relationship with God. All soul development is a development in love, either Natural Love or the Divine Love that is given by God. (These two kinds of love will be discussed more fully in Chapter 2 and 6.) It is your soul development in love that determines your happiness and your attractions to events and situations in your life. The level of love in your soul also determines the condition of your spirit body and the youthfulness of your physical body.

It is the soul and not the personality that goes through a journey of ascension back to God to pure light. The soul instinctively seeks to return and reunite with God even if the mind does not consciously make us aware of our soul's desire. If you focus on the soul and not on the physical body or the intellectual mind, then your soul's journey home to a place of perfected love will accelerate. This means that ultimately your suffering will end, and your soul will reside in a place of eternal bliss.

## THE SPIRIT BODY

There is an aura and an existence of an electromagnetic field around every object in the world, including you. The spirit body is also known as the etheric body or aura, and your entire physical body is surrounded by it. It is attached to the soul by a golden cord and to the physical body by a silver cord. It is an invisible energy field controlled and affected by the condition of the soul. The size of your spirit body or aura is unique to you and dependent on the state of your soul condition. Even though most people cannot see the spirit body with their human eyes, they can sometimes feel it. But there are some people who are sensitive enough to see someone else's aura.

Your spirit body is the etheric map for the physical body and holds the complete template of the physical. Every cell in the physical body has an etheric counterpart. The spirit body has the same structure as the physical body, including all the anatomical parts and all the organs. The etheric body creates the grid on which the physical body grows and is responsible for the vital transfer of information and life-force energy from the universal energy field. It also acts as a filtration system. Universal energy filters down through the soul to the spirit body to the physical.

At death the spirit body detaches from the physical body, but it remains attached to the soul and still has a mind. The spirit body is still living and thinking after death. It is important people take note that their spirit body reflects the true condition of their soul. Even if you had good genes, the body of an athlete or a "beautiful" supermodel, that is of no consequence if you did not do deep soul work or release negative emotions such as anger or hatred from your soul while you were alive, because the contents of your soul will be degraded and your spirit body will look deformed after death. For some people it can be a shock to see their damaged spirit body once they cross over to the Other Side.

## THE CHAKRA SYSTEM

Running through your aura or spirit body are many layers known as subtle energy bodies, auric layers, or meridians. Our soul is an energetic system where emotions are running constantly. These emotions cause energy meridians in the body. These subtle energy bodies are controlled by the soul and the emotions contained in our soul. There is a synergis- tic relationship between each of the auric layers or energy bodies. Each one is interconnected so what affects one layer, affects the others. These distinct layers of energy are intimately connected to what is known as a *chakra system.*

The chakra system is made up of seven subtle energy points and distribution centers that draw in divine life-force energy from the uni-

verse and distribute this vital energy to the physical glands and organs
in the body through both the bloodstream and nervous system for
optimum health and well-being. A chakra is a center of activity that
receives, assimilates, and expresses life-force energy. *Chakra* is a Sanskrit
word meaning wheel, so chakras are sometimes referred to as "wheels
of light." These "wheels" spin at a particular rate, frequency, and vibration. The seven chakra points are where the energy meridians intersect
in our body.

As energy is distributed through your body via the chakra system, it
cycles energy from the soul to the spirit body and eventually into the
physical body. When your energy body is functioning properly and
your chakra points are balanced, open, and spinning at a similar rate to
each other, your energy flows smoothly, and your physical body is
healthy. Unfortunately, most people have some chakras which are over-
active and others that are shut down or underactive, so the energy
cannot flow equally to all parts of the body. This causes blockages and
imbalances. As we saw earlier in this chapter, these blockages and
imbalances are caused by negative emotions which, in turn, cause your
body's vibrational frequency to slow down, so your energy becomes
heavier. As your frequency lowers, toxins accumulate and your cells
start to become dense, diseased, and old.

The seven major chakras are located along the spinal column—
starting at your perineum (the region of the body below the pelvic
diaphragm and between the legs) and going up to the top of your head
at your crown. There are more chakra points in the spirit body above
and beyond your head and your body. There are chakras behind each
of your joints, in your palms, hands, and soles of your feet. As you
progress spiritually, you become more aware that you have many more
chakras with different functions, but for now we are going to focus on
the seven well-known chakra points nearest to your body. These affect
you most directly. This is why we often hear the number seven mentioned in many spiritual texts.

Each of the seven chakra points have a different function, vibrational
frequency, musical note, and color that corresponds and is connected to
specific physical tissues, organs, muscles, and areas of the nervous system through different meridians. Color is a living energy. It is a prop-

erty of light. Light is an electromagnetic energy produced by the sun in different wavelengths. The electromagnetic nature of color cooperates with the energetic structures of a human body, strengthening or suppressing their vibrations. Different colors give off distinctive wavelength frequencies, and these frequencies have different effects on physical and psychological functions. We all emit color, have our own unique energy system, and have organs that have different vibrational patterns.

As you have already read, sound is vibration. Each chakra vibrates at a different frequency, from the lowest/deepest/slowest frequency at the root to the highest/fastest at the crown—with each chakra having its own sound, just as it has its own color. The musical notes of the chakras start at middle C at the root and get higher as you move further up the body. The entire chakra system creates an octave. Music and sound, good or bad, influence us and impact our energy systems because we adjust our energy to match that of the music. Each song or musical note we listen to has its own particular frequency.

Below are the seven different chakra points on our body with their corresponding functions, locations, vibrational notes, and colors. Each of the seven musical notes and seven colors corresponding to the chakras has emotional and physical issues attached to it. Each of the seven chakras represents a definite set of desires that correspond to a particular element; therefore, understanding the seven chakras offers a way to balance desires and lead to a happier life while fulfilling personal destiny. When you have gained the necessary information and the healing tools to keep the chakras balanced and healthy, then you can allow the song of your soul to be heard.

The **first chakra**—the **root** chakra—is represented by the color red and the musical note middle C. It is located at the base of the spine. It forms your foundation, connects you to the physical earth, and provides you with your feelings of security and survival. It is the basis for human existence in the physical world. It roots the subtle divine consciousness in the material life. Emotionally, this is the chakra where we connect with the family in which we were raised. It reflects a person's connection with his or her mother and with Mother Earth. Ideally this chakra brings us health, prosperity, security, and dynamic presence.

The **second chakra**—the **feeling** center—is located in the abdomen, lower back, and sexual organs and has an orange hue. Its musical note is D. This chakra is associated with the parts of the consciousness concerned with food and sex. It connects you to your emotions and your sexuality. Ideally this chakra brings us depth of feeling, sexual fulfillment, and the ability to accept change.

The **third chakra**—the **power** chakra—is located in your solar plexus and is represented by the color yellow and the musical note E. It rules your personal power as well as your metabolism and digestion. It is the emotional power center where you take control and authority of yourself. When healthy, this chakra brings us energy, effectiveness, and nondominating power.

The **fourth chakra**—the **heart** chakra—has green as its color and its musical note is F. It is located at the center of the chest. This chakra is associated with the heart and the blood circulatory system as well as the lungs, the thymus gland, and the entire chest area. It is associated with love, relationships, compassion, and healing. A healthy fourth chakra allows us to love deeply, feel compassion, and experience a deep sense of peace and centeredness.

The **fifth chakra**—the **throat** chakra—is your communication center. Its color is blue, and its musical note is G. It connects you with the right to speak and the power of truth through the spoken word. The throat chakra helps a person express truth fearlessly. When this chakra is clear and open, it allows us to be powerful communicators in the world.

The **sixth chakra**—the **third eye**—is located at the forehead between the eyes and is represented by the color indigo and the musical note A. It is associated with developing your intuition, self-realization, and a balanced state of mind. It helps to focus the mind. When healthy, the third eye allows us to "see" clearly with our innate psychic powers.

Finally the **seventh chakra**—the **crown** chakra—is located at the top of the head and is represented by the color violet and the musical note B. It connects you to God's consciousness, to learning about your spirituality, and to the spiritual realms. It is associated in the body with the pineal gland and the cerebral cortex as well as with consciousness

# The Chakra System

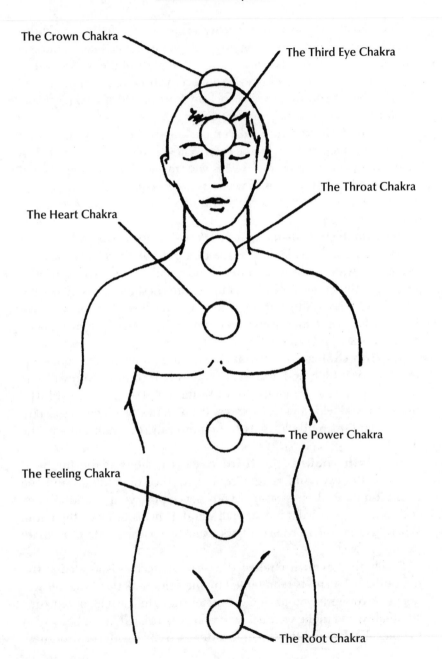

The Crown Chakra

The Third Eye Chakra

The Throat Chakra

The Heart Chakra

The Power Chakra

The Feeling Chakra

The Root Chakra

and spiritual enlightenment. When developed, this chakra brings us knowledge, wisdom, understanding, spiritual connection, and bliss.

## THE MIND (SUBCONSCIOUS MIND)

Your spirit body also has an etheric mind that communicates with your brain. This part, known as the subconscious mind, is associated with your mental and rational world. It is filled not only with different thought patterns and belief systems but also religious and social attitudes that have been programmed into you since childhood. It can easily become contaminated with negative forms of thought that often appear logical to the thinker. These thought forms are directly affected by the emotions in your soul which, in turn, affect the physical body. A healthy mind is interested in learning and serves you well, but if your emotions are negative and you have a lot of emotional injuries, you will feel pain and have negative thoughts. When your emotions are healthy, then your mind is healthy and thinks in a positive way, keeping your body in a healthy state. The mind of the spirit body continues to function after death, communicating telepathically with other spirits and with humans on earth.

## THE PHYSICAL BODY

The physical body, also known as the material human body, is denser than the etheric body because it is designed to feel both pleasurable and painful sensations. It is energy materialized into solid matter. Your physical body is attached to the spirit body by a silver cord. At death, the cord attached to the spirit body detaches from the physical body so that this body no longer receives a stream of life-force energy and information. This causes physical death.

Your physical body has a brain that communicates directly with the mind of the spirit body (the subconscious mind). The brain is the main computer of your physical body; it sends messages to parts of your body so they can fulfill necessary bodily functions and actions. The brain controls the body either by activating muscles or by causing secretions of chemicals such as hormones and neurotransmitters. As the human soul purifies and expands its level of consciousness, soul–to–soul communication takes over while the mind and brain become less dominant and less controlling. You begin to communicate through feeling, which is the only true form of communication. Your memories and intelligence are actually in the soul. When the soul and spirit body disconnects from the physical body at death, the brain dies.

## How the Three Bodies Affect You

When you understand the basic flow of energy through your soul and your spirit body to your physical body, you can begin to understand that your physical body—the level of matter itself—is the result of hidden causes taking place in the soul. Many healers are concluding that disease can be identified in the soul and spirit body before it manifests in the physical. In fact, the term *dis-ease* literally describes the imbalance in your energy systems. As you become "ill at ease" with your thoughts and feelings, they will eventually manifest as some form of disease or disorder in your spirit body and physical body.

The cycle of energy through your systems changes the state of the subtle energy field around you, especially when you become imbalanced and your feelings change. If you feel hatred, shame, or fear, that energy will flow from your soul into your aura, which will lower your vibration level and damage your physical body. As the vibration of energy lowers and the quality of the energy gets denser, it slows the flow and causes blockages. We record every thought and feeling in one of our seven chakras, and they become lodged there until they are released. This slows down the chakras spin rate. When your energy vibration gets slower and your body gets denser, your cells and body move further away from their naturally high and light vibrational state which is the state of perfected love. This causes your cells to age and die. So if you want to change your spirit body and your physical body, you have to change the contents of your soul.

## How Do You Stay Young?

Now you have the full picture to enable understanding of the workings of your physical body, your soul, and spirit body. You can begin to reverse the aging process and heal the years of harm you have unwittingly done to yourself. Hopefully, as you look in the mirror, the invisible has become visible now so that you can approach the rejuvenation of your body in a new way.

But where do you begin your healing process? How do you start to tap into the eternal fountain of youth? It is simple; you have to purify your mind, body, and soul. You have to embark on a program of spiritual, mental, physical, and emotional detoxification. You have got to say goodbye to the old in order for your cells and your soul to be reborn.

You need to set about restoring your youthful beauty and vitality by beginning a journey back to a place of perfected love, which is the highest of energy vibrations. This state of perfected love is known as becoming at one with God or *at-onement* with God. You reach this high level of energy frequency by clearing your Qi, unblocking your chakra system, cleansing your mind, your spirit body, your physical body, and your soul, especially, of all the emotional, physical, mental, and spiritual toxins that have accumulated in your system since childhood. You need to take yourself back to the beginning, to your foundation, when you were once a pristine soul with pure energy and no false beliefs, negative thoughts or feelings.

As I said at the beginning of this chapter, spiritual masters treat their bodies as sacred temples—a place to house their souls. To maintain their body temples and keep them looking golden, shining, and brand new, they dedicate time to cleaning and honoring the soul inside.

If you want to begin the process of healing and age reversal, then you, too, need to become a master and learn how to treat your body as a sacred space, worshipping not just the outside temple but the inside of your soul.

"But," I hear you panic, "how can I become a spiritual master? I'm an ordinary person. I can't possibly reverse all the harm I have done to my body when my life has been so hard? It's too late to start now because too many years have gone by. I'm over forty; I feel overwhelmed. I need a quick fix; I don't have the time to do all this work."

Believe me when I say that you can create a new body that self-replenishes, does not self-destruct, and stays healthy, vibrant, and young. You can become your own healer, dermatologist, dietician, fitness trainer, and spiritual guru. There are already thousands of ordinary people doing this process. You can become a spiritual master in your own right, especially if you make the purification of your body, mind, and soul an important part of your daily schedule.

Once you have decluttered your system and removed all of the emotional toxicity, energetic density, and the physical damage, you will go through a metamorphosis. A transformational alchemy will occur in your cells. Your DNA will recode and change as your body returns to a state of "lightness" and well-being. All the blockages will be released, and your energy will start to flow properly through your chakra system again.

Your body will vibrate at a much higher frequency—the same frequency as the field of universal love. As you raise your vibration rate, your body will become more nourished in its own being. It will transform into a light body by allowing less trapped matter to manifest and allowing light to enter so you are not so solid. It is at this state of high vibration that you will tap into the eternal fountain of youth.

From this ageless, sacred place you will have an abundance of energy. Your aura will become brighter and more expansive; you will start to radiate light from your eyes, and your face will transmit your beautiful energy. Other people will begin to notice your change; they will feel drawn to your light and your pure, loving soul. You will become the superbeing whom God intended you to be—a vessel of youth, vitality, love, and true beauty.

So be assured that you can naturally redesign yourself, but it is going to take some commitment, some reorganization of priorities, and an oath to declutter. But do not be overwhelmed; the process can be easy if you simply dedicate a small amount of your busy day to staying pure and balanced. When you change your priorities and your outlook, not only will your face have a spiritual facelift, but your entire life will be uplifted and forever changed for the better.

Now that you have full understanding of the powerful destiny that lies ahead, you can start your natural health and beauty program today. Follow the seven steps of purification in this book, and stay open to the spiritual truths that you read in each chapter even if they feel strange at first. Your soul will soon awaken to truth again and organically start its healing journey back to pure light and love.

Remember, your goal should not be to create a perfect physical body. Your goal should be to stay focused on your destinations of finding the real you—your authentic self—and of reaching a state of perfected love in your soul. It is only at the level of soul purity, love, and authenticity that your body will function at the highest of energy vibrations and will heal itself naturally. From this place of perfected love, your life will also transform.

Go be a spiritual master; go claim what is rightfully yours—your health, your beauty, and the best years of your life.

## • *Exercises for Energy Awareness* •

The following exercises will help to develop a sensory gift and awareness of energy. Please do not get discouraged if you do not get immediate results. It may take some time to develop an ability to read, see, feel, and sense energy. As you work your way through your purification process over the next few weeks and months, you will clear emotional blocks, your body will become filled with more light, and you will become more sensitive to your own energy and the energy of others. Just keep practicing and you will soon see results.

### Exercise 1: Learning to Sense Energy

This exercise will build your awareness of the energy all around you and heighten your ability to "read" your own energy field and that of other people.

- Rub your hands together until you create friction and you feel your hands heat up. Hold your hands out with palms facing each other. Feel the energy between your hands as you try to push them together. You will become aware of your own energy field or aura. You will begin to realize that your energy field acts just like a magnet. It will repel things that do not have the same frequency or attract things that are the same frequency.
- Walk around your house and feel the energy of the different rooms. Walk into the room where you spend the most time. Feel your energy imprint that has filled your space. Pick up some of your personal possessions and feel the energy of the objects. Your personal energy field has been absorbed by these objects.
- Does your spouse have a private work space? Now go into his/her room and feel that energy. Feel the energy of his/her possessions. Do the two rooms and the two sets of possessions feel different?
- If you have children, go into their rooms and feel their different energy. If you do not have a partner or children, visit an array of friends and feel the different energy in their houses. You will see that each friend has a unique frequency and the energy will vary. Is the energy light and bright or is it dense, depressing, and heavy? Feel the reaction in your body as

you enter each individual's room. Focus especially on your solar plexus, heart chakra, and your "gut" feeling. Remember how those areas in your body feel.

- Keep practicing this exercise so you can reprogram yourself to understand that you, everyone, and everything are composed of energy and that some energy is light and positive while other energy is dense and negative.

**Exercise 2: Seeing Energy**

Some people can actually learn to see energy. You might already have the gift of second "sight."

- Ask a friend to stand against a white wall. As you look at your friend, do not try to focus; just let your eyes relax, and you may be able to see a rainbow of colors above his or her head or round the hands and body. If you see colors, you are seeing the spirit body or aura. Are the colors vivid and powerful or dark and barely visible? Does this aura expand a long way or is the energy field thin and dim?
- Ask a friend to read your aura/energy field while you stand against a white wall.

**Exercise 3: Changing Your Energy with Music**

Music can be a useful medium to help you change and clear your energy field. Sound in the form of music, musical notes, or chanting can be used for chakra balancing. Repetition of sound supports bringing the body, mind, and soul into a meditative state, where healing occurs and creates a continuous vibrational environment. The frequency of music affects our own energy frequency because we adjust our energy to match that of the music. Your energy will change from dark to light with the click of a CD play button. Visualization with the associated chakra color while using sound can deepen and amplify the healing experience. Sounds may be soft and gentle; they do not have to be loud. You do not have to sing to sound the chakra notes; you can sound them silently or aloud. Follow these exercises and you will see.

- Put on a selection of music. Listen to a happy, upbeat song and see how your energy feels. Then put on some loud rock. Now play a slow sad song and feel how your energy frequency changes.
- You will feel your energy change from a high light frequency to a low energy. Feel how your body, especially your heart chakra and solar plexus, responds to the music. When you feel sad, heavy, and bad, remember that feeling in your body. When it feels good, light, and bright, remember the feeling in your heart chakra and solar plexus. These are your "Yes" or "No" beacons. Keep changing the music so you can fine tune your ability to "read" your energy beacons and determine which energy feels good and what feels unhealthy for you.
- Sing, hum, or silently sound each chakra note for up to five minutes each, starting at the root and working your way up the body. Musical notes can also be chanted as part of a sound meditation. Focus on the chakra as you sound the associated note. The more you allow the musical note to resonate throughout your body, the deeper the healing affect.
- Buy a Tibetan singing bowl. Its sound will resonate through your chakra system. They create a wonderful, healing sound.
- Buy a set of wind chimes to clear the energy inside and outside your home.

**Exercise 4: Changing Your Energy with Color**

- Color is energy and the energy of color affects our frequency. Your energy changes as you wear different colored clothes or when you paint a room a particular color. Practice feeling how your energy changes as you tune into the color of your clothes or enter a colored room. Color can be dense or light, either giving energy or absorbing energy. Feel how the dense color of black absorbs energy and how white purifies and lightens your energy field. Color can brighten your mood, soften you, and make you feel stronger or put you in a bad mood. Blue soothes and protects while red is passionate and makes you feel more powerful; green calms the body and releases anger as orange brings joy and helps you heal from grief and loss; yellow is used for mental stimulation; pink opens the heart to unconditional love, and purple connects you to your spirituality and brings success into your life. If you are in need of more power in your energy field, then wear a red sweater; if you want to connect to your femininity and find love, wear a pink shirt, or if you want to connect further to your higher self, then put on a purple dress.

**Exercise 5: Unblock Your Energy Meridians**

- You can book an appointment with an acupuncturist to rebalance and unblock your energy meridians. Acupuncture will help you relax and help energy flow smoothly through your chakra system so your body can stay young and healthy. Acupuncture works directly with the body's energy or Qi. Acupuncture practitioners believe that all illnesses are a result of the natural flow of energy through the body becoming stuck, depleted, or weakened. Acupuncture benefits the rebalance of Qi through treatment of specific acupoints related to symptoms. Treatment is effective in removing these energy obstructions.
- You can also visit a reflexologist who will massage the energy points on the soles of your feet. These points correlate with different organs in your body. You can also massage the energy points of your own feet at home to save time and money.
- You can balance your chakra system by visiting a Reiki practitioner. Reiki (pronounced Ray Key) is a combination of two Japanese words *rei* and *ki* meaning universal life energy. Reiki is an ancient laying-on-of-hands healing technique that uses the life-force energy to heal and balance the subtle energies within our bodies.
- You can practice the art of hands-on healing with friends. Place your hands on a friend's shoulders. Close your eyes and imagine sending energy from you into his/her body. Feel energy move down from your crown chakra through your body, down your arms, and out of your hands. You should start to feel your hands heat up and your friend's shoulders should start to feel warm. This is how many hands-on healers cure people of aches, pains, and illnesses. Ask your friend to tell you how he/she is feeling at the end of this exercise; then ask your friend to place his/her hands on you so you can experience an energy healing.
- Please note to be careful whom you allow to place his/her hands on you or send you energy. If his/her soul is not purified, then you do not want your energy field contaminated with less than the highest quality of

energy. Ensure that any practitioner you seek is a highly qualified Reiki expert or acupuncturist who understands the importance of emotional clearing and the difference between the spirit/etheric body and the soul.

- As your soul and energy field purifies, you will no longer need or have any desire to see a healer or outside source to help you heal or to make your body look younger. You will be your own self-healing, self-replenishing mind, body, and soul. This should be the end goal of your spiritual purification program.

**Exercise 6: Learning to Exercise with Energy**

Eastern martial arts techniques and exercise programs such as Tai Chi and Qi Gong will help you further understand and work with the energy of the universe and the energy of your body. The exercises harness the Qi or life energy force. They are slow and magnetically charged movements that are gentle, yet provide a very strong sense of Qi. Just lifting your hands along the front of your body can send a wave of heat and magnetic sensation (Qi) moving through your entire body. Buy a Tai Chi or Qi Gong DVD to practice at home or take a class in your local community.

- Tai Chi, also called Tai Chi Chuan, is a noncompetitive, self-paced system of gentle physical exercise and stretching. To do Tai Chi, you perform a series of postures or movements in a slow, graceful manner. Each posture flows into the next without pause, ensuring that your body is in constant motion. Through proper breathing and movements that should be taught by a Tai Chi master, you will be able to achieve a harmonious state. Tai Chi can also be used for meditation and other health purposes. Tai Chi can also help you defend yourself in times of trouble by teaching you how to deflect the intentions and energy of your attacker.
- Qi Gong (ch'i kung, chi gong), China's ancient system of energy medicine, consists of exercises and meditations that stimulate the flow of Qi, life energy. It is the philosophy and practice of aligning breath, physical activity, and awareness for mental, spiritual, and physical health as well as the development of human potential. As a spiritual art rooted in Taoism, it deepens awareness of self and nature as it creates a wonderful feeling of peace and harmony.

**Exercise 7: Learning to Scan Energy**

Learning to feel the energy of objects can be very useful—especially if you have lost your keys or your glasses. You can learn to tune into the object whether it is in your near vicinity or somewhere else. You will "feel" exactly where it is by sensing its energy field.

- Hold your glasses or keys and tune into the frequency. Remember the feeling of the energy of the keys and how you feel in your "gut" when you tune into them. Now ask your friend to hide the keys or glasses. Try and tune into the energy of the object. Feel the sensation in your solar plexus as you try to scan the room for your keys or glasses. You will soon learn to scan a room for something you have lost, and you will know whether or not it is in the room by realizing if you can feel its energy. This exercise will help you deepen the ability to read your own Yes/No energy beacons.

**Exercise 8: Tuning into Other People's Energy**

Just as you can learn to scan objects, you can also learn to scan people's energy fields. Practice this scanning technique on different people, such as strangers you meet or people whose hands you shake. When you learn to scan a person's energy field, your body will tell you all you need to know about his/her soul condition and intentions, no matter how they look or what they are saying.

- Drop your attention down into your heart chakra and solar plexus instead of listening to the thoughts running through your head. These thoughts are often affected by outer appearances and can be biased or deceptive about the actual truth of the person standing before you. You will start to feel your own Yes/No beacons and a sense of good or bad energy in your intuitive center. You will feel nauseous as you tune into someone with negative energy who is unhealthy for you and just the opposite as you scan something or someone full of light energy, goodness, and love.

**Exercise 9: Sending and Receiving Energy**

This exercise will help you understand the power of energy and how far your energy travels.

- Think of a friend and send him/her your loving energy. See how quickly you receive an e-mail or a phone call from that person. He/she will say, "I was thinking of you." Of course he/she was because your energy was sent out into the universe and directed at someone so he/she immediately felt your energy and presence.
- Remember that energy travels through time and space. You will usually hear from someone a day or two after you have sent that person a thought or feeling if he/she is emotionally connected and energetically open. Try it and see.

**Exercise 10: Crystal Rebalancing**

- You can also experience different energy vibrations with colored crystals. You can use them as a supportive tool to help accelerate your deep soul work. They help unleash emotional blockages. The power of the crystal is not a hocus-pocus New Age myth. Many people have been healed through the powerful energy of crystals. They have been spoken about in ancient Indian texts and Chinese medicine as well as being referenced in the Bible. Throughout time, many cultures have understood the magic of crystals. They are a God-given gift from nature with remarkable healing properties.
- Each crystal has its own specific function and frequency to heal different areas of your body and to purify your chakra system. Crystals absorb your negative energy and replenish your body with their healing energy frequencies. Tune into a crystal, and your energy will change to match its. You can place crystals on your body at different chakra points to rebalance and heal your chakra system.
- Crystals such as jade, topaz, amethyst, citrine, rose quartz, aquamarine, tiger iron, and garnet can help you sleep, heal your heart, clear your aura, and give you extra strength.
- You will learn more about the power of crystals and their specific healing

qualities for different areas of your body throughout the book. But I recommend that you purchase a book on crystals so you can learn more. There is a whole array of crystals, and they all have different healing properties.

- Crystals can really change the energy of a room. Place some rose quartz in a bowl by your bed or a large amethyst on a coffee table. You could also place a piece of opal on your desk to create a good atmosphere at home and at work. Crystals not only change the energy of a space but also make great home accessories. They look very colorful and decorative.
- If you place specific crystals under your pillow at night, your energy will shift to match the energy of the crystal. Any emotional blockages will surface while you are sleeping.
- Carry a crystal in your pocket or wear a crystal as an attractive piece of jewelry round your neck.
- You can also make crystal elixirs if you place a crystal in a glass of water, leave it in the refrigerator overnight and drink the water the next morning. You can also meditate while holding crystals.
- Regularly clean your crystals by first dusting them with a dry clean cloth; then place them in warm salt water. Once you have soaked your crystals, put them outside in the sun for fifteen minutes. This will keep their energy field strong and will cleanse away the negative energy the crystals may have absorbed from you and your surroundings.

# 2
# Eradicating Facial Wrinkles

*A quiet mind speaks the loudest.*
**Mae Chee Sansanee Sthirasuta**

When we were young, we left the house without an ounce of makeup on and ran around naked. We enjoyed our day without a care in the world. But as we hit our teenage years and the first break out of blemishes appeared, we ran screaming back into our bedrooms. Paranoia set in; we felt that our lives were over and we were never going to be able to show our faces again. From those first moments of teenage angst, our struggles continue the older we get. Wrinkles set in like railway tracks spreading across our foreheads, telling the tale of each difficult year of our lives.

## WHAT CAUSES WRINKLES?

Facial wrinkles become more of a problem with every year that passes. The face is the most exposed area of the body—an open book for all to see, revealing hidden secrets and shedding light on a person's real age. But seemingly, the days of worrying about wrinkles are finally over. The marketplace is full of products and procedures that all promote a smoother, ageless, and wrinkle-free face. Women are spending much of their time and money at dermatologists, willing to bear the discomfort of Botox needles and an extortionately high bill. As the old sayings go: "You have to suffer to look beautiful. What's a little bit of poison, if it means my wrinkles are no longer visible? So what if I cannot fully animate my face anymore? It is actually a good thing I have no facial expressions, otherwise they will know that deep down inside I'm really depressed."

But what so many people do not realize is that the expensive potions and painful procedures they are paying for are only a short-term fix. These remedies are a cover-up and do not get to the root cause of why we get wrinkles in the first place. As soon as one wrinkle is erased, another appears, and the endless cycle of wrinkled skin continues. But what if I were to tell you that you could naturally erase your wrinkles without any expensive dermatological visits or spiders' poisons paralyzing your face? What if your wrinkles could fade away, one by one, with following a safe, simple program that starts with one change inside of you?

Often we hear people say "every line on my face tells a story." This is true. Your life is mapped out on your face: the laughter, the struggles, the joy, and the pain. Your forehead is creased because it tells the world that your life story has been full of stress, conflict, and tension. Your face is a reflection of your inner dialogue. It shows all the angst taking place inside of your head. All the constant thoughts, discussions, and arguments that run twenty-four hours a day through your stressed-out mind are reflected by your worry lines as you try to figure out solutions that deal with daily conflicts and the aggravating people, who literally get in your face. This blocks the flow of energy around your face. The Chinese would say you have blocked *Qi*.

Look closely in the mirror; each line on your face has been caused by a repetitive facial expression. As you repeatedly pull your face to express your tension, irritation, and stress, a deep energetic imprint is left in your facial tissue. Over time those repetitive motions leave a buildup of energetic imprints that generates wrinkles, deep crevices, and worry lines created by an internal reaction to an external person or event.

How you feel on the inside influences the thoughts in your head and the lines on your forehead. If you have negative emotions inside of your soul, your thinking will be negative. You repeatedly display those negative thoughts and feelings. Then your eyebrows begin to knit together as you ponder how to resolve your latest conflict or dilemma, and the vertical crease between your eyebrows also gets deeper, more prominent, and harder to fix. Back to the dermatologist you trek every month to pack your lines with toxic fillers that eat away not only at your time and your money but also at the skin on your face.

A forehead of wrinkles shows you have a troubled and cluttered mind; you are out of balance and using up too much mental energy. Intellectuals are especially prone to overthinking and facial lines. They are focused on the mind rather than their heart and soul because they are avoiding their emotions. People living in the mind praise logic, and they dismiss or minimize feelings. Conversely, people living in the soul understand that when they are connected to their true feelings, everything becomes completely logical and understandable. A person living in the mind separates feelings and emotions from thoughts and logic while someone living from his or her soul knows that honoring feelings and emotions is the best way for a person to remain in a state of harmony and clarity.

Remember that the condition of your soul impacts the energy of your spirit body and your subconscious mind. This, in turn, impacts your physical body, your material brain, and your cells. Remember also that a feeling originates in your soul and creates a thought in the subconscious mind of your spirit body. This, in turn, communicates with the brain leading you to speak words through your mouth or communicate through actions. What you feel—you think about—you do and become. Your feelings and thoughts create your reality. If you have pain and suppressed negative emotions inside of your soul, then your thinking will also be negative and so will your actions and words.

Each thought form and feeling will either add highly vibrating energy that will run smoothly through your chakra system and keep your cells light, vibrant, and alive, or will feed low, dense negative energy to your body that blocks your chakra points. The dense energy of your thoughts especially affects the sixth chakra, your third eye, which is situated on your forehead. When you live in the mind, your energy will stagnate, build up in your temples, and manifest as heavy lines or worse still, blockages of energy in the third eye can lead to tumors of the pituitary or the pineal glands. Excessive energy also builds up in the brain due to the modern-day overuse of cell phones. Cell phones are being linked to brain tumors due to too much heat, energy, and radiation which mutates brain cells. People who are constantly on the phone are trying to keep their minds busy to avoid their deeper emotions.

Living a life from your mind rather than from your soul can cause all sorts of stress, health, and personal problems in your life because your egoic mind controls you. It lies and defends you at all costs. It lives in fear of being defeated and exposed. It is overly attached to the external and material world because it desires power and control. Then it tells you all sorts of negative stories about yourself and other people.

At the physical level and at a lower soul condition the steps required to communicate are subject to many stages, and as a result, there is greater potential for many errors to occur. As you grow in love, you become less dependent on your intellect and develop your capacity to assimilate truth through your soul.

"But how do I keep my mind quiet and stop negative thoughts from entering my head?" I hear you ask. "I'm not a spiritual leader; I don't live in a monastery where life is peaceful. I have to deal with work, my partner, my mother-in-law, and my kids. It is going to be impossible for me to erase my wrinkles, especially when the world is in such a terrible state."

Albert Einstein once said, "Peace cannot be kept by force. It can only be achieved by understanding." Inner and outer peace can only be achieved by gaining knowledge. If you want to erase your wrinkles, smooth out your forehead, and learn to clear your mind so you can reduce stress and become more peaceful inside, then it is vital that you gain more knowledge about your mind, body, and soul.

## How to Clear Wrinkles

It is going to take courage and emotional honesty to clear the stag-

## Communication at the Physical Level

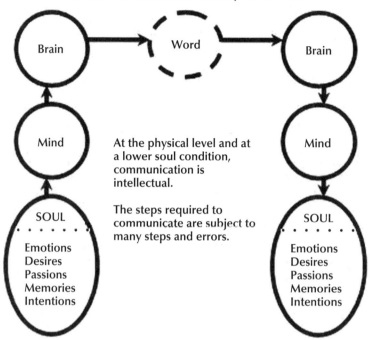

At the physical level and at a lower soul condition, communication is intellectual.

The steps required to communicate are subject to many steps and errors.

## Communication at the Soul Level

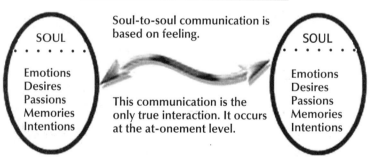

Soul-to-soul communication is based on feeling.

This communication is the only true interaction. It occurs at the at-onement level.

A feeling originates in your soul and creates a thought in the subconscious mind of your spirit body. This, in turn, communicates with the brain leading you to speak words through your mouth or communicate through actions. Your feelings and thoughts fill your body with either light positive energy or negative dense energy. As you clear your soul and spiritually evolve, you will stop communicating through the mind and brain. You will develop soul-to-soul communication abilities. All soul communication is based on feeling.

nant energy that has built up on your forehead. While you are applying your face cream, desperately trying to erase your wrinkles, you need to ask yourself these questions: "*Who* or *what* is getting in my face?" and "*Why* is this person or event staying on my face?" Once you have answers to these two important questions, you can start to release your wrinkles.

As you look at your face, you will know deep down what caused each one of your wrinkles. Was it your finances, your neighbors, your car, your family, or your romantic relationship? If you want to clear your face, you are going to have to look deep inside of your soul and get to the root of your emotional conflict. Each wrinkle guides you to confront deeper emotional injuries from childhood that are the causes of your turmoil. These injuries created every single line on your face.

Many New Age and Eastern spiritual teachers mistakenly try to teach their followers to stay mentally peaceful by deliberately changing their thinking. But changing your negative thoughts will be only a temporary fix; they will keep returning if you do not permanently clear the emotional reasons that created the thoughts and your stressful reactions in the first place.

In Chapter 3, Energetic Liposuction, you will learn powerful techniques to help you access and release childhood emotional injuries so you can lose weight and clear all your negative emotions from your soul. As you clear emotions, your body will get lighter and your thoughts will change from negative to positive. Your mind will no longer lead and dominate. As your soul clears and expands in its ability to love, your soul intelligence will likewise grow. As you have read, your memories and intelligence are in the soul. You will receive vast packets of information and begin to communicate directly from your soul to another soul rather than through your mind and material brain. All soul communication is based on feeling. This is the only true form of communication. It occurs when you are at-one with God. Soul-to-soul communication will cause you to shift your focus from your head to your heart, which will reduce the energy build up in your temples and thereby reduce your wrinkles.

For the rest of Chapter 2, you will gather more vital information to erase your facial wrinkles and ease your stressed-out mind. At the end of this chapter, you will also learn practical exercises and an array of natural remedies to keep your mind healthy and to clear the wrinkles that you have already accumulated. But how do you ensure that they do not return? Even if you change your negative thoughts and emotions, you will most likely be able to only momentarily reduce your stressful reactions because the belief systems conditioned and programmed in your mind will still be the same. That is why erasing your wrinkles can only be permanent if you fully clear your mind of all disharmonious societal, family, and religious beliefs.

## CLEARING FALSE BELIEFS

No matter our current beliefs about God or religion, we all need a guiding light, a goal, or a target—something more perfected than we are to lead us down the correct path to happiness. God created a myriad of laws to help educate your soul and bring you back into a state of peace and harmony. These universal laws help to remove conflict inside of you and lead you to a place of perfected love. They guide you back to mental and emotional balance and show you how to live a life free from stress and suffering.

Your mind is associated with your mental and rational world. It is filled with different thought patterns and beliefs as well as religious and social attitudes that have been programmed into you since childhood. If these belief systems are in harmony with God's universal laws, your soul condition will be healthy; your thoughts will be pure; you will be nonreactive, and your life will be peaceful and free of pain. But if your belief systems are error based and disharmonious, then your thoughts and feelings will cause stress, and you will continue to pull tense, angst-ridden facial expressions.

If you can reprogram your mind so that your belief systems stop creating destructive, unloving thoughts and feelings towards you and other people, then much of your conflict will end. For example, many women use Botox or synthetic fillers to smooth out the deep, vertical dividing line between their eyebrows. What they do not know is that this vertical crease can be erased naturally because it is not caused by old age but by a belief system that separates them from others and creates divisions in the mind.

Your forehead crease, the dividing line on your face, is a reflection of the divisions inside you. The reason the heavy line is becoming more and more prominent every year is because you are conflicted. You always knit your brows together, thinking about dilemmas you are having with a particular person or situation. You battle to make a decision. You are torn in two because of your disharmonious belief systems.

Destructive belief systems were ingrained in you from a young age when you were first told that the world is divided into dualisms such as boys and girls, rich and poor, good and bad people. These dualistic belief systems began separating you from other people. They also made you hide the darker side of you—those negative emotions filling your soul such as hate, fear, shame, jealousy, or anger. You feared you would be judged and that you would not be loved if you revealed the truth about how you were really feeling so you began to hide parts of yourself.

It can be hard to face the divided parts of yourself and heal your divisions with other people. People tend to defend themselves, blame others, and try to hide their dark side because they feel guilty or ashamed—they suffer from feelings of unworthiness and self-hate. They have not been taught that God loves them unconditionally, and because their parents have not loved them unconditionally, they judge and punish themselves harshly. They then judge and punish others harshly, too. Their shadow selves stay hidden for most of their lives. But if you resist looking at your dark side and your negative emotions, your secret feelings become even more extreme and create an even greater divided self. Not only does that prolong the pain and conflict in your life, but it also builds up a vertical crease on your face.

This crease grows deeper because of the conflict between your intellect and your emotions. This conflict can become so extreme that it causes a war inside you—a battle between the mind and soul. It can lead to the violent mood swings seen in people with bipolar disorder. The intellectual mind tries to suppress the true emotion underneath, but before long the emotion comes surging to the surface in displays of not only extreme highs and lows but also erratic behavior.

If you can learn to embrace your shadow self and the divisions inside of you caused by your childhood emotional injuries and understand that both your good and bad sides as well as your negative and positive emotions are the whole of your being, you can then start to transform your soul. This transformation will also help you clear your conflicted mind.

As you learn to love and embrace all parts of your being unconditionally and to bring "light" to your "darker" side by purging your negative thoughts and emotional injuries, your wounds will start to heal and you will become a whole person. Your darkness will no longer be locked away in a secret compartment. When you shine light on a shadow, it disappears. The more you bring light and expose the disharmonious dark feelings buried deep inside of you, the more your negative emotions and thoughts will disappear and so will that vertical crease dividing your face. Ironically, you will stay mentally healthy and ensure that you never have a spell in a mental hospital if you lose your suppressive, controlling, and dominating mind and reconnect to your true emotions instead. As you connect to and follow the logic of the emotions in your soul, then your mind will rebalance and get quieter.

## GOD'S UNIVERSAL LAWS

God wants to free us all from mental, emotional, spiritual, and physical suffering; therefore, God designed a series of universal laws as a feedback system to help guide us. This divine system is not meant to punish us but rather to bring us back to a state of harmony and perfected love. But many people find they do not want to live by someone else's laws. They do not want to give up their personal truth. They do not understand that the real meaning of personal truth is actually what God sees as the truth about you. Divine Truth is what God sees as the ultimate truth of the universe. Divine Truth will never accommodate itself to the beliefs of men. Men have to accommodate their beliefs to Divine Truth.

Deprogramming your set of belief systems may be difficult at first, especially if you have followed a very specific religious or spiritual practice or do not believe that God exists at all or have unresolved childhood issues around authority. You may dig in and say, "My beliefs are my beliefs, and there is no changing them." Your parents may have been very stern or you went to a school that had strict rules so you may say, "No one is going to tell me what to do." If you could only remember that sometimes laws, especially God's divine laws, have been created to benefit and protect you rather than restrict, punish, or repress you, then this might not be so difficult to accept.

If you are resistant to change, then remember that nothing in life is permanent. How many times have you been adamant about your opinion and then a few years later done a 180-degree turn when you believed something completely different? How many times has a scientist proven a certain law of physics and then had to refine his work when new information came to light? The world is always changing, just like the change of seasons in nature; the only permanent thing is impermanence itself and the truth about God's universal laws. If you hold on too tight to your beliefs and cling to something that is not in harmony with God's Truth because it seems too painful to accept that you might be wrong, you will continue to feel only pain and stress in your life. Often our personal truth is based on fear and is in error from God's perspective.

When you realize that what you have been taught and believed all your life is not the whole of God's Truth, it can bring up a lot of grief about your life. What if you have lived many years following belief systems that ultimately turn out not to be true or to have been misinterpreted? The fear of feeling grief about how you have been lied to or how different your life would have been if you had known the whole truth may be so intense that you resort to anger and refuse to allow any new knowledge to enter. But God's knowledge and wisdom is infinite—an absolute truth—the Divine Truth that has no finality. New information is coming to light all the time. You should not allow yourself to stay locked in the darkness of a stubborn, fearful mind. Every day God is trying to awaken us to something new about the universe and ourselves.

That is why I hope you can stay open to the new information in this chapter. If you can allow Divine Truth to enter and be open to investigate the possibility of a false belief, then perhaps your life will change for the better. As you continue to read this chapter, allow yourself to investigate how your current belief may need expanding. Permit yourself to identify, experience, and release your fears and also feel, experience, and release the underlying causal emotion that is blocking you from Divine Truth. Truth is often felt to be "painful," but in reality, only error is painful. If you feel pain when you read the following truths of God, then it is not because you are hearing truth but because you are releasing errors that you have been carrying for all your life. If you can let your knowledge be eternally progressive and can align your personal truth with God's Divine Truth, your life will be filled with greater peace, clarity, and understanding. As the saying goes, "The truth will set you free."

## LAWS OF NATURAL LOVE AND DIVINE LOVE

If you understand God's universal laws, you will understand everything that happens in your life. Everything happening in and around you is a result of either living in harmony or disharmony with these laws. If you understand and embrace this truth, you can ease your physical, spiritual, emotional, and mental suffering. When we feel pain, we are in error and out of harmony with God's laws; when we feel joy, peace, and love, we are living in harmony with Divine Truth and Love.

God created many universal laws as a divine guidance system, but most people have ever heard about only a few. They understand the physical laws, such as the Law of Gravity, the Law of Thermodynamics, and the Law of Electromagnetism. Throughout the centuries scientists have studied the physical laws and have proved how they operate on physical and metaphysical matter. Most people know that their life is governed by physical laws, especially that of the Law of Gravity which allows them to walk on the planet.

But few people understand God's higher spiritual laws of *Natural Love* and *Divine Love* even though these are the most important ones they need to learn. The laws of Natural Love and Divine Love transform the soul and help end suffering permanently.

Gaining knowledge and wisdom about God's spiritual laws is the most important gift people can give themselves because it is the soul-based laws that affect your level of happiness. These laws are higher than the physical or metaphysical laws which do not operate on the soul so therefore do not affect how you feel. As an adult, our personal pain and long-term suffering are the result of personally breaking God's spiritual laws. All God's laws are loving in their operation and have loving consequences upon the soul; they always operate whether you are aware of them or not.

The reason most people follow only the physical laws is because they feel an immediate, painful impact on the body such as a broken leg or arm if they go against gravity and fall out of a tree. What they do not realize is that breaking the higher spiritual laws of God creates an automatic penalty on the soul that also immediately impacts the condition of the spirit body and ultimately the physical body.

When you awaken to God's higher laws, you will become aware of all your illusions and will learn the truth about life. These laws will not only change the way you think and feel but will also change your reality and perception of the world around you, which will further impact your thinking. You cannot control people or stop life's difficult situations, but you can change how you react to them by following God's universal laws.

Following is a brief overview of God's laws of Natural Love and Divine Love. You can apply these laws to your current spiritual practice or religious belief system. There are hundreds of other universal laws, but I have selected only the main laws that directly affect and govern your inner and outer life. If you can follow them in your life, you will reduce your stress, your facial tension, and therefore, your wrinkles. For life to exist and continue to exist, the universe must remain in a state of harmony. Therefore, each law God creates or has created results in a completely harmonious universe for all of creation. These divine laws confirm that God is not, as many people teach, a punishing God but rather a loving God because all of these laws help to end suffering and lead us all back to a place of perfected love.

# 1. NATURAL LOVE LAWS

Natural Love laws are moral or spiritual laws governing and operating on the soul. They are higher laws than the physical laws such as the Law of Gravity. Portions of these laws are reflected in most religions and spiritual practices, but often they are incomplete. Very few people on earth fully understand the laws of Natural Love even though they govern our enjoyment of life.

The laws that people have heard of are the moral commandments dealing with killing, stealing, or committing adultery. But what many do not understand is that even if people do not physically break a moral law by taking action and killing, stealing, or cheating but they think about killing, stealing, or cheating, then they have still broken God's spiritual laws of Natural Love because of their innermost thoughts and feelings. This will create an instant emotional penalty on the soul, which will degrade the soul condition and therefore, the spirit body and physical body. The purpose of the penalty is not to punish but rather to correct the person and bring him or her back into a state of harmony with the universe, the true state of happiness. God does not exact the penalty for the violation of the law; the law does it itself.

Your soul condition is significantly influenced by Natural Love laws because they show you not only how to love yourself spiritually, emotionally, and physically but also how to love other people. Natural Love laws help to develop the love that comes from inside the human soul, from within you. Natural love exists as an emotion within your soul and can be given to and felt by another human. If you are in disharmony with these laws, you will feel unhappy. If you are unhappy, then God's divine system is showing you that a law of love is being broken. There is an emotional penalty on the soul that is causing you pain; you probably learned the wrong things about love as a child.

Examples of Natural Love laws are: the Law of Free Will, the Law of Attraction, the Law of Cause and Effect, the Law of Compensation (also known as the Law of Karma), and the Law of Desire.

## The Law of Free Will

The Law of Free Will is one of the most important of God's laws of Natural Love. It is a gift from God that allows us to choose or do anything we desire. By acting on your free will throughout your life, especially as an adult, you have been able to gain knowledge about who you are and why you are here. The Law of Free Will allows us to act in harmony with anything that is truthful (loving) or in error (unloving). When we love ourselves, we always enable our free will whether others agree with our decisions or not. If you follow this law, you never suppress the exercise of your own free will even if other people want you to. You will never suppress feeling and experiencing your own emotions or doing what you desire even if it is in complete disharmony with Divine Truth and Love. But you recognize that if you exercise your free will in disharmony with God's laws, you will suffer consequences and feel an emotional penalty in your soul.

If you go against your free will, it shows you that you do not love yourself; you have an addiction to "being loved" caused by a painful childhood emotional injury that makes you feel unworthy. Likewise, if you react negatively or try to stop someone else's free will because he or she is not conforming to what you want, then you are out of harmony with God's laws. This stems from a need to be in control and a desire to avoid recognizing your deeper emotions.

## The Law of Attraction

The Law of Attraction means that our thoughts and feelings co-create our reality; what we think about we create; what we feel, we attract into our lives. The energy of our thoughts and feelings manifests into a physical reality.

Our Law of Attraction is God's messenger of truth, showing us what needs healing in our soul. The soul is a powerful magnet, and our feelings are the main basis of the Law of Attraction. Emotions are electromagnetically charged so they attract or repel into our life other electromagnetically charged things in the surrounding universe. The soul condition determines every single thing that comes into your life and all future experiences through the Law of Attraction. You can only change your Law of Attraction by changing your soul condition. If you experience a negative event, it shows there is something that you must resolve within yourself. Once you have cleared any emotional injuries from your soul, then you will be able to manifest anything positive your heart desires.

The only people who do not have any Law of Attraction are children. Because children do not have free will at birth, they have no Law of Attraction until they are older. They are subject to their parents' Law of Attraction which means that anything which happens to a young child is caused by suppressed emotions in the parent. When parents clear their emotional injuries and addictions, their child will automatically heal.

## THE LAW OF CAUSE AND EFFECT

This powerful law means that what you sow, you will reap. Every action that you do creates a positive or negative reaction. What you send out into the universe comes back to you and has an effect. Everything that has happened in your life and your physical body is the result of some cause. If you only attempt to change the effects and never address the cause, then the effects will continue. You need to treat the cause; otherwise your Law of Attraction will never change. If you follow this law, you will never blame another person or try to avoid the emotions created by events and situations in your everyday life. You need to look at what soul condition in yourself prevents you from being in harmony with the Law of Cause and Effect. It usually derives from a fear of feeling your childhood emotions. When you do not address the cause of your feelings, then much of your time and energy will be spent trying to control other people and avoid your own painful emotions. This will cause you to feel frustrated and exhausted.

## THE LAW OF COMPENSATION/KARMA

This law revolves around the instant penalties the soul incurs if you are unloving and break the laws of Natural Love. The Law of Compensation is different from the Law of Cause and Effect because it operates only on the personal level of your own soul and does not affect anyone else. The effect of breaking the law is man's punishment inflicted on himself because of his memories and awareness of the unloving actions he has taken against himself or another. The Law of Compensation cannot be avoided under any circumstances because it was created to help a person develop in natural love.

The only way the Law of Compensation can be stopped is to release our painful memories. Some people live for many years in great pain before they receive relief because they cannot forget what they have done. As the painful memories leave, the person will suffer less. He or she will be free from the penalties of the law, but it could take years of suffering until the feeling of freedom arises.

The most powerful way to relieve people of their painful memories is love. This love comes in the form of remorse, sorrow, and the desire to make amends for any harm caused. But until love is awakened, a person usually cannot feel remorse, regret, or the desire to made amends. Once people feel remorse, the penalty is eradicated, and the soul is restored to a pure state.

## THE LAW OF DESIRE

Ask and you shall receive! This law means that what you desire, you get. If you have a passionate longing and desire in your soul for something, you can manifest it. If you develop and allow a passionate longing for anything, whether that thing is harmonious or disharmonious with Divine Truth and Love, you will receive it. Your own desires and passions are paramount to your soul progression. Your soul has incarnated to fulfill its desires so if you do not follow your soul's desire, you will experience pain.

The results of this law create either pleasurable or painful experiences in your life. You can have a variety of desires that range from romantic love or material things to being a mother or a business owner, yet the highest desire is a passion for God's Divine Love. If your desires are in harmony with God's Truth and Love, your soul's desires will bring you great happiness and joy. If your desires are out of harmony, then the consequences can be harmful. The saying "Be careful what you wish for" is true.

## 2. DIVINE LOVE LAWS

The Divine Love laws operate upon the soul at the highest level and allow infinite soul progression. They affect the overall condition of the soul and can override Natural Love laws. These laws govern our connection with God and assist the transformation of our human soul into something divine and immortal. Few people on earth have ever heard of these laws even though they determine our universal existence. Most people feel these laws are purely religious and unscientific in nature and therefore invalid. None of these laws can be understood intellectually; they can be understood only emotionally at the level of soul perception.

Examples of Divine Love laws are: the Law of Repentance, the Law of Forgiveness, the Law of Divine Truth, and the Law of New Birth.

### THE LAW OF DIVINE TRUTH

Divine Truth is the absolute, infinite truth of God; without it love cannot be complete. Divine Truth can only enter the soul emotionally; it is felt rather than intellectually understood. Divine Truth does not compromise, even to keep the peace. Many religions and New Age circles teach portions of Divine Truth, but most distort Divine Truth by intellectualizing and theorizing about it. God's Truth is not personal truth, although personal truth can become absolute truth if we grow towards God. When you follow the law, you speak, feel, and live in harmony with God's Truth at all times, never withholding truth, no matter what the consequences are or what anyone else feels. Emotional truthfulness is the most loving act you can do to heal both yourself and others. Divine Truth is essential because it is only the truth that truly sets you free.

### THE LAW OF FORGIVENESS

This law shows there is no reason to refuse to forgive in any situation—forgive others just as God forgives you—freely and immediately. If you do not forgive, then your soul will be filled with resentment and anger, which will cause physical, mental, emotional, and spiritual harm. Forgiveness is not intellectual but emotional. When you have forgiven, there will be no emotional charge or emotional signature left inside of your soul. This means you will not remember the event or what a particular person did to you. When an emotional signature is released, its physical manifestation has no foundation and is, therefore, neutralized. The Law of Attraction will show you when forgiveness is complete because you will feel no more anger or resentment towards the people who have hurt you. You will not avoid or fear meeting them unless they choose to repeat their harmful actions.

## THE LAW OF REPENTANCE

The Law of Repentance operates only on the human soul and nothing else. It is a Divine Love law that is higher than the Law of Compensation. Repentance is a feeling of deep grief and sorrow and is a desire to right the wrong. When we truly awaken to the error of our ways and want to make amends, then we become remorseful. Then the law kicks in automatically, and the error is removed from your soul. If you do not repent, you will still feel the painful memories of your harmful actions, which will make you suffer and affect your Law of Attraction. Once you become repentant, the emotional penalty clears and your Law of Attraction changes.

## THE LAW OF MERCY

The Law of Mercy activates to show lenience to a person who has caused harm. People should learn to forgive automatically so that they do not cause harm to themselves or their environment, but mercy should be shown only once a person shows remorse. Mercy is a similar quality to God's Grace. It is only appropriate to demonstrate mercy when a person feels sorry for his or her actions.

Even though that person is automatically forgiven by God, it is wise to allow the Law of Compensation or Karma to operate, and only when a person displays a desire to make amends is mercy appropriate. If the Law of Mercy activates before a person has repented, then he or she will not heal and not see the error of his or her ways. He or she will not learn how to become harmonious with God's Love. If the person does not feel remorse, then he or she will probably do the same action again.

## THE LAW OF THE NEW BIRTH

The Law of the New Birth is the transformation of the soul from the human into the Divine. This transformation can happen only when the soul purifies and receives Divine Love from God. Without the new birth, eternal progression is impossible for the human soul. Divine Love is the love that comes directly from God. It exists as an emotion within God's soul that can be given to and felt by any human. Divine Love cannot be given through the intervention of another human or a spirit. It is not the love state of the human soul at incarnation nor is it a state of perfected natural love. Divine Love can be infinitely received by the human soul, but it can flow only when the soul is in harmony with Divine Truth. Divine Love can also only come into the human soul when the human so desires and longs for it to enter. This happens through prayer. When God's Divine Love enters the soul, it helps increase a person's level of happiness; the soul expands and transforms the human soul into a divine human. At this point, the person obtains knowledge of his or her immortality and reflects God to mankind.

Now that you have learned the different types of God's spiritual laws, you will hopefully be able to start feeling and thinking in a new way. You are armed with a new outlook on life, and from this vantage point you can reduce the stress in your life and the worry lines it causes. Following God's divine laws will lead you to a more harmonious place of perfected love, the highest of frequencies. It will slow your aging process, heal your body, and keep your life running smoothly.

## LEARNING TO BREATHE

Another tool to help you stay relaxed and stop you from thinking too much and acquiring worry lines is learning to breathe properly. I cannot stress enough how important it is to learn to breathe. When you breathe deeply, you have an eternal tool. You cannot stop your thoughts from coming; they will come and go through the day, but you can control your breathing. Your breathing will support you throughout the day and keep you connected to your soul rather than focused on your mind.

Even though taking a deep breath is the first thing we instinctively do when we are born, most people do not breathe properly. They run around, stressed out, holding their breath. They do not breathe deeply from their bellies, and the result is that they are not getting enough oxygen circulating throughout their face and body to nourish all their cells. When they focus on breathing properly, their facial muscles are relaxed. It is through the practice of breathing that we are able to be in the present moment of each inhalation and truly relax. Each breath brings fresh energy into the body, and the exhalation releases toxins along with depleted energy. Deep breathing provides a feeling of oneness of body and breath rather than a simple autonomic nervous system function.

Just as you have to remember to eat and drink regularly throughout the day, so you should check that you are focusing on your belly and breathing deeply so that your stomach is pushed in and out and your face is relaxed. This should be an essential part of your daily health and beauty regime.

As you read this book, check to see how deep your breathing is and how much tension is being held in your face. You probably clench in one or all areas of your face and take shallow breaths from your chest rather than deep breaths from your stomach. Learn to breathe deeply, in and out, and loosen your facial muscles. Unclench your jaw, a major area for holding tension. Now stretch the skin on your face; open your eyes wide; imagine chewing sticky toffee with your mouth, and stretch the creases in your forehead. Next, unfurrow your brow and make sure you allow your face to be bright and open.

Any time you sit at your computer, watch television, or read, check your breathing and the tension in your face. Shallow, tense breathing is going to be a life-long habit that you will need to break. You must become conscious of your facial habits and your breathing until your mind, body, and face have been reprogrammed and you naturally relax.

## LEARNING TO MEDITATE

Your level of relaxation and deep breathing can be taken even further if you can take a moment out of your day, either first thing in the morning or last thing at night, to meditate. Meditation allows your mind to rest completely and to empty itself of all thoughts. It also helps relax the facial muscles. It can help you feel calm, happy, content, and relaxed or emotionally present. Both spiritual masters and scientists say that meditation brings measurable changes in brain regions associated with memory, sense of self, empathy, and stress. As you rest and replenish the mind when you meditate, you will experience many health and beauty benefits.

You may, at first, feel resistant to sitting for long periods of time, but if you can just take five to fifteen minutes a day to close your eyes, you will rest your facial muscles completely and fill your body with positive, life-enhancing energy. This will smooth out your forehead and give your body a surge of vitality.

Meditation opens your third eye, the sixth chakra in your chakra system. This is the chakra that helps you become self-realized, develop intuition, and balance your mind. As your third eye opens, your sixth chakra point will become unblocked, and your stagnant energy will start to flow smoothly away from your forehead and out of your system. Meditating and opening your third eye will help you break free of old belief systems and negative thought patterns. As your intuition develops, you will "see" more of life's truths. You will learn to observe your inner life with your inner third eye. This new clarity and vision will help further remove the vertical crease on your forehead while balancing your mind, body, and soul.

If you feel you are too busy, you can meditate even if you are not sitting in a chair with your eyes closed. You can meditate throughout your day with every breath, no matter what you are doing, as long as you breathe correctly. You can meditate when you are doing any of your daily activities: walking the dog, washing up, ironing, fishing, cleaning, gardening, showering, creating a picture, molding a sculpture, or playing music. As long as you concentrate on breathing deeply from your stomach instead of your chest, your mind will become quiet and focused on the present moment, and you will replenish and nourish your body with healing energy.

Gentle exercise can also be considered a form of meditation. A gentle meditative walk outside in nature is a powerful stress reliever. As you read in Chapter 1, an exercise practice, such as Tai Chi or Qi Gong, can be especially beneficial to promoting a peaceful state of mind.

Tai Chi is sometimes described as "meditation in motion" because it promotes serenity through gentle movements—connecting the mind and body. The main goal of Tai Chi is to teach you how to deal with stress by relaxing your mind and calming your body. During Tai Chi you focus on movement and breathing. This combination will help you to melt away your stress, anxiety, and tension.

As you progress with clearing your soul of negative emotions, your need for meditation will slow. Once you are at one with God, it will eventually cease. This is because you will not have emotions in your soul creating negative thoughts, actions, or events. (You can read more about the Law of Attraction in Chapter 5.) Your mind will be very peaceful because there will be no stress or conflict in your life. If you need to meditate, that is a sign you still have negative emotions to process deep in your soul. But completely purifying your soul, reaching a place of perfected love, and becoming at one with God where you are free from suffering, takes time. It is here that meditation can be a useful support tool until your emotional injuries are gone.

Be aware that you should not use meditation to disconnect from your emotions. Meditation is not meant for emotional avoidance. You cannot clear your soul through clearing your mind. You clear your mind by clearing the emotions in your soul. If you feel that you cannot get through your day without meditating, then you are addicted and are avoiding your emotions. You are fearful of feeling your emotional pain. Do your emotional clearing work first, and then sit down to meditate. You can do that by focusing on refilling your body with fresh energy. Purge your negative emotions while inhaling and thereby replenishing pure, higher vibrating energy from God's universe. Eventually, your soul will be clear; your deep breathing will be constant, and your inner and outer world will be peaceful

## PRACTICAL TOOLS

Now you have the inner tools to help you remove your facial wrinkles, but there are also practical steps you can take to support your internal process to ensure you have a youthful face.

The next step to creating a wrinkle-free face, alongside of your deep soul work, the learning of God's laws, proper breathing, meditation, and a gentle exercise program, is to remove makeup, oil, and environmental contaminants from your skin.

The cleansing of your skin should not be just a morning ritual. At night, make sure you remove your makeup and cleanse properly before you go to bed. It is very damaging for your skin to get into bed leaving makeup and environmental grime on your face while you sleep. Use a natural cleanser or a natural, oil-free makeup remover. Once your face is clean, moisturize with a natural face cream that is oil free. Ideally, your face cream should contain alpha lipoeic acids, alpha hydroxy acids, amino acids, Vitamin A, C, and E, peptides, and peptide complexes. Try also to find a natural cream containing beeswax or zinc oxide, which stimulates the renewal of collagen, diminishes fine lines and wrinkles, and increases firmness as well as elasticity. Zinc helps boost elastin (the skin's protein) production. Do not rub or pull your face while applying your face cream. Rubbing stretches your skin and can promote sagging and wrinkles. You should also apply a natural sunscreen over your moisturizer. Another great tip is to sleep on your back instead of your front so you minimize creasing your face. If you press your face to your pillow, you will experience increased puffiness in the morning.

Exfoliation is important for removing dead skin cells from the skin's surface. There are many homemade exfoliants you can make that slough off dead skin cells and create smoother, more radiant skin. Baking soda is a very effective and popular exfoliant. Its natural abrasive texture combined with its ability to neutralize acidity makes it an excellent choice for an exfoliating process. Three effective face masks may also be made from just oatmeal, avocado and sesame oil, or ground almond and yogurt.

Many natural beauty experts offer a natural facelift whereby they work away your wrinkles with a deep facial tissue massage or employ advanced technology using light and sound waves. I recommend that you treat yourself to a professional facial. It is important to pamper yourself. It is an act of self–love. But ensure that you go to only a highly regarded, certified practitioner who uses nontoxic organic products. If you cannot put it in your mouth, do not put it on your face. If you cannot spell or understand the ingredients, do not allow anyone to put them on your skin. Do not get addicted to these professional procedures and merely start to focus on the outside of your face again. Remember to put your main focus on the emotional cause of the "who," "what," or "why" that is getting in your face.

This commitment to using natural products should extend to your makeup line. Most makeup products are made of synthetic materials that can severely damage your skin and the health of the cells in your body. There are many new mineral eye shadows and foundations available in the marketplace that nurture the skin and infuse it with non-drying, beneficial minerals.

Facial toning acupuncture can also be very effective and leave you with a radiant complexion. It stimulates the blood flow and facial muscles, improves your skin texture, and increases the collagen in the face. Facial toning acupuncture began in China over eight hundred years ago and was used to maintain the beauty of the favorite concubines. With hundreds of years of history behind it, facial toning acupuncture is a tried and tested holistic treatment. Microdermabrasion and facial peels are also effective treatments for blemishes, wrinkles, and uneven skin pigmentation.

If you cannot afford to pay for a professional treatment, do not worry; you can still treat yourself to a daily pampering. At the end of your busy day, I highly recommend that you give yourself a facial massage every night as you sit and watch television. Work your fingers through the skin of your forehead to smooth away the deep crevices and wrinkles. Remember that you are unblocking stagnant energy and creating a flow with your hand movements. Use your index fingers or knuckles to mold the skin deeply, upwards and out with circular motions. Move the deep energetic imprints up and away; let the old stale energy unclog from your facial tissue. Do not forget your neck. So often we concentrate on only the face, but your neck should also be part of your morning and nighttime moisturizing regime. Massage moisturizer into your neck with upward strokes so you do not pull the skin. Make this nurturing, deep tissue facial and neck massage the perfect ending to your stressful day. Use organic oil when you massage your face and neck so that you do not "burn" the skin. Vitamin E oil is very healing for the skin. Coconut oil is also effective. It contains rich antioxidants and nutrients, helps fight bacteria, and naturally diminishes wrinkles. Coconut soap is a powerful facial cleanser, and coconut water can cure acne scars. This is due to coconut water's cleansing and toning effects on the skin. These natural products are relatively cheap in comparison to the many expensive antiwrinkle creams in the market place that are full of harmful chemicals.

Proper nourishment and supplementation are also the keys to healthy skin, healthy brain function, and a peaceful state of mind. The food in your kitchen is the perfect solution to skin and mood problems. If you are to protect your skin and keep yourself emotionally and mentally healthy, it is important that you eat a diet high in antioxidants and rich in nutrients. Fruits, whole grains, and vegetables are highly nutritious and keep the body as well as the brain functioning properly.

These following types of foods should be the main ingredients in your diet. Avocados contain niacin (Vitamin B3) which is especially important for healthier skin. Niacin is anti-inflammatory so it soothes irritated blotchy skin. You can both eat avocado regularly and prepare it as a weekly facial mask. Eating fruits such as mangoes, which contain Vitamin A, helps to maintain and repair skin cells. Vitamin A is an antioxidant that fights free radical damage that can prematurely age the skin. (You can read more information about free radical damage in Chapter 5.)

A handful of almonds every day can provide 100 percent of your daily need for Vitamin E, which, as you read, contains powerful healing properties for your complexion. Cottage cheese, Brazil nuts, salmon, or cod contain selenium, which is an essential antioxidant mineral for the skin. Citrus fruits such as grapefruits or oranges supply 100 percent of your daily allowance for Vitamin C, which fights skin damage, prevents wrinkles, and produces collagen, the structural protein in your skin.

Even oysters fight acne because they are rich in zinc.

Mushrooms are rich in riboflavin (Vitamin B2.) Riboflavin is involved in tissue maintenance and repair. It also improves blemishes caused by skin disorders such as rosacea. Wheat germ is a good source of biotin, which is crucial to skin health. Finally, cucumbers, especially cucumber skin, can greatly improve your complexion. Cucumbers have an abundance of antioxidants and silica, which can leave skin soft and smooth. They can be used in a face mask or as a toner to tighten pores.

Hyaluronic acid is a popular antiwrinkle remedy. In 2003, the FDA approved hyaluronan injections for filling soft tissue defects such as facial wrinkles. Restylane is a common trade name for the product. Hyaluronan injections temporarily smooth wrinkles by adding volume under the skin with the effects typically lasting for six months. Nowadays you can find facial serums with hyaluronic acid and many body lotions that contain it.

Hyaluronic acid can also be accessed through safer natural food sources. Soy is a great vegetable option because of its tendency to increase levels of estrogen in the body which, in turn, increases levels of hyaluronic acid. Tofu or soy bean curd and edamame, soy beans in their original baby form, are the most versatile soy food. Soy milk, soy ice cream, or soy yogurt are other options. Hyaluronic acid can also be sourced from sweet potatoes and other starchy roots. Low levels of hyaluronic acid have been found in individuals with low zinc and magnesium levels. You can source magnesium from a variety of magnesium rich fruits such as apples, bananas, strawberries, tomatoes, avocados, pineapples, oranges, papayas, melons, peaches, and pears. Legumes such as kidney beans, pinto beans, black-eyed peas, and lentils are also rich in magnesium.

Glutathione is an important nutrient needed to give skin a radiant glow and to defy the aging process. It makes pores finer so your skin becomes smoother and clearer. It also controls acne and prevents acne marks. Glutathione is an amino acid found in every cell of a living organism. It is the ultimate antioxidant because it protects the body from a multitude of diseases and conditions. But as we age, our glutathione levels are depleted due to exposure to air pollutants, stress, drugs, smoking, or food chemicals that damage our cellular systems.

Glutathione can be taken as a supplement, or it can be found in foods, such as broccoli, cauliflower, Brussels sprouts, and cabbage. Various herbs such as cinnamon and cardamom have compounds that can restore healthy levels of glutathione. The high amount of selenium in Brazil nuts can also increase glutathione levels. Coenzyme Q10 (CoQ10) is also a beneficial supplement. CoQ10 is an antioxidant compound made naturally by the body that protects cells from free radicals and promotes healthy cell growth. As we age, our levels of CoQ10 begin to deplete. It is one of the few antioxidants to have shown effectiveness as an external topical product. Many face creams, foundations, cleansers, masks, overnight skin care nourishments, and daytime moisturizers containing pure forms of CoQ10 are becoming popular. They have shown almost immediate results with skin tone, elasticity, and age spots. Foods that contain CoQ10 include soybeans, sesame seeds, corn oils, sardine, mackerel, tuna, herring, peanuts, pistachios, walnuts, adzuki beans, and hazelnuts.

Other necessary supplements are selenium, which reduces the risk of sunburn and promotes an even skin tone, and Vitamin C, which keeps the skin firm and maintains the collagen in our skin.

Taking a high grade B complex vitamin and liquid trace minerals will also give your body extra support. They will not only keep your skin healthy but your brain alert and functioning properly so that you do not get so stressed. Folic acid, also called folate, is a B vitamin that is often deficient in people who are depressed. The mineral chromium is also important for brain health. It is becoming very popular as a natural remedy for depression. Unfortunately our soil has become severely depleted of this vital trace mineral, and therefore, it is also lacking in our food source. We should take extra chromium everyday in supplemental form.

Not only is chromium needed for healthy brain function and curing depression, it is also the main mineral responsible for the conversion of sugar into energy. Many people are diabetic, not just because they are overeating and consuming an unhealthy diet but also due to the fact that chromium is no longer present in the food source. The inability to convert sugar in our body causes not only insulin disorders and glucose intolerance but also depression and other psychotic behaviors. The

sugar literally shocks the brain, severely impacting its ability to function properly and creating emotional disturbances.

Hypoglycemia is also a hidden epidemic causing low blood sugar
issues, mood swings, and sugar cravings. The brain becomes starved of
glucose and goes into shock; sometimes comas occur because the body
is unable to regulate sugar levels. Most alcoholics are hypoglycemic;
they crave sugar. Many people with mental health problems are also
hypoglycemic. Hypoglycemic women exhibit symptoms of depression
when their sugar is low and men are known to become violent and
angry. I believe that millions of people are being unnecessarily locked
up in mental hospitals and given mind-numbing drugs because of a
simple lack of proper nutrition for the brain and because of blood sugar
issues. Many prisoners are also being locked up for violent or angry
behaviors due to low blood sugar disorders. All alcoholics, mental
health patients, and those under arrest should have tests for hypoglycemia and diabetes before they are either committed to a mental institu-
tion or incarcerated in jail. Organic foods and natural supplementation
for the brain should play a mandatory role in the justice and mental
health systems.

Stress drains the body of magnesium. Magnesium helps to produce
serotonin, a mood-elevating chemical within the brain that creates a
feeling of calm and relaxation. Epsom salts, which is hydrated magnesium sulfate, is considered to be a natural stress reliever. When dis-
solved in warm water, magnesium sulfate is absorbed through the skin
and replenishes the level of magnesium in the body. The salt draws
toxins from the body, sedates the nervous system, reduces swelling, and
relaxes muscles. The experts believe that bathing with Epsom salts at
least three times a week helps a person look better, feel better, and gain
more energy. Magnesium ions also relax and reduce irritability by lowering the affects of adrenaline.

Studies have also linked depression with insufficient intake of omega-
3 fatty acids. Fats make up 60 percent of the brain and the nerves that
run every system in the body. So it stands to reason that the better the
fat in the diet, the better the brain. The average American brain is getting
enough fat, but it is not getting the right kind of fat. In countries such as
Japan and Taiwan who have higher fish consumption, which is a good

source of the omega fatty acids, the depression rate is ten times lower than in North American. Postpartum depression is also less common.

The body needs two kinds of fat to manufacture healthy brain cells which act as the message senders and prostaglandins which are the messengers. These are omega-6 fatty acids found in many oils, such as safflower, sunflower, corn, and sesame oils, and omega-3 fatty acids found in flax, pumpkin seeds, walnuts, and coldwater fish, such as salmon and tuna. Most important to brain function are the two essential fatty acids: linoleic (or omega-6) and alpha linolenic (or omega-3). These are the prime structural components of brain cell membranes and are also an important part of the enzymes within cell membranes that allow the membranes to transport valuable nutrients in and out of the cells. Our bodies cannot make omega-3s on their own, so we must obtain them through our diet.

Flaxseed is an especially powerful natural antiwrinkle agent. Our bodies use the essential fatty acids (EFA) contained in flaxseed oil to metabolize vitamins, produce hormones, and protect us at a cellular level. Our skin has a fatty layer made up of these acids and additional fats. The more omega-3 fatty acids you have in your body, the stronger the layer of fat will be around the skin cells, meaning that your cells (and your skin) will be plumper. When you plump up the skin, the appearance of wrinkles diminishes. Fatty acids also dilute sebum and unclog pores that otherwise lead to acne. Sebum is an oily substance secreted by the sebaceous glands in mammalian skin. Its main purpose is to make the skin and hair waterproof and to protect them from drying out. An excess of sebum, however, can make the skin or hair oily. When you use omega-3s as part of your regular diet, you will notice that your skin complexion will begin to look cleaner, fuller, and smoother.

The importance of nutrition for skin health is discussed in greater detail in Chapter 5. You will read more examples of antioxidant nutritious foods and natural supplements that stop premature aging and keep your body functioning optimally. There is no need for dangerous procedures, synthetic mood-altering drugs, or antiaging products. Nature provides for all of our beauty and mental-health needs.

## CONCLUSION

All people can achieve a peaceful state of mind and wrinkle-free face, if they stop thinking and start feeling, if they heal their divided self, learn to live in harmony with God's laws, eat healthily, take proper supplementation, exercise gently, and learn to breathe properly.

No matter what you do throughout the day, no matter how positive you stay, you are always going to encounter situations that may be stressful and difficult, or you may come in contact with unhappy people who personally attack you. You cannot control how other people are going to react to you, but you can use how you react to them as a guide to your inner and outer healing. Your reactions are a spiritual guide to show you the condition of your soul. The more you release your emotional injuries and purify your soul, the less you will react—and the less you will get attacked.

If you turn your eyes inwards and observe only your own feelings, thoughts, words, actions, and behaviors instead of critically watching other people on the outside and focusing on whether what they are doing is right or wrong, then you will progress rapidly.

If you stop attaching to the outside of yourself and look deep inside, you will discover a whole new, exciting inner world. If you can find the courage to shine a light on your shadow self, you will, in fact, come to enjoy living from your soul and discovering your feelings. You will realize that your innermost feelings have great power. If you follow the logic of your emotions instead of a cluttered, ego-driven mind, you will realize your inner world dictates your outer reality. This awakening will not only erase your facial wrinkles but will empower you and dramatically transform your life.

So keep following God's universal laws of Natural Love and Divine Love, and open yourself up to new belief systems. God's guidance system will bring you back to a state of peace and harmony. Each of the laws will be covered further throughout the book. By the time you have finished reading *Spiritual Facelift*, you will be well versed in God's spiritual laws and free from all the false belief systems that cause you conflict, unnecessary mental stress, and facial wrinkles.

Do not get upset if you sometimes fail to live by all of God's laws. It takes time to reprogram your mind and embody a totally new, stress-free way of feeling, thinking, and living. Remember that the whole goal of this spiritual health and beauty program is to move you towards a place of perfected love. Do not judge yourself if you fail at the beginning, for that would be unloving to you. A lack of self-love will lower your energy vibration and age your cells. God already feels you are perfect, no matter what stage you are on your spiritual journey.

## • *Exercises for Eradicating Facial Lines* •

**Exercise 1: Change Your Language**

- Learn to change your language from saying "I'm thinking" to "I'm feeling." Ask people how or what they are feeling rather what they are thinking so they connect to their real emotions and not their intellectual mind. Be an example, share with people how you feel about something rather than what you think. This will help you to start to live a soul-based existence. Remember, emotions are the seat of the soul.

**Exercise 2: Releasing False Belief Systems**

- Write a list of all of your belief systems. What do you believe determines good and bad? What do you believe is right and wrong? Who do you believe is good and who is evil?
- Write a list of the ancestral belief systems that have been passed down through your family line. How many of these do you live your life by?
- Write a list of societal, religious, and political belief systems that cause you to feel divided from other people. What are your views?
- Compare all of these different belief systems with God's laws of Natural and Divine Love. How do they differ? Put them in two columns:
  i) Belief systems that are aligned with God's laws that make you feel free, happy, connected, and peaceful within yourself and with other people (unconditional love, free will, living passions and desires, abundance, and joy.)
  ii) Belief systems that are out of alignment with God laws that make you feel stressed, divided, in conflict, and unhappy (pain, conditions, expectations, lack, struggle, suppression, exploitation, abuse.)

**Exercise 3: Clear Emotions around Authority**

- If you are going to give up your personal truth and live a life guided by God's laws, you need to clear emotional injuries around authority.
- Think back to your childhood with your parents and your school days, and feel your emotions around any negative experiences with authority.

Were you punished unfairly? Did the rules you had to follow cause unnecessary suffering? How were you punished when you broke your school rules or your parents' rules? Feel and release the painful emotions so you can accept God's loving guidance system.

**Exercise 4: Clear the Vertical Crease**

- Write a list of all of your good traits. Are you unconditionally loving and kind, patient and wise? Now make a list of your negative traits. Are you impatient, stubborn, selfish, manipulative, unbending, rude, or mean?
- Look at the list of things that you feel are not so good about you. Instead of denial, sit with it and embrace the truth. Do not let your ego try to defend you. The more you hide things, the bigger they become inside. Face this "shadow self" inside of you. Feel your negative traits and the root cause of why you have them. Once you determine the cause of why you feel and behave in a certain way, then you can start to release your negative emotions and heal your shadow self. (See Chapter 3 to learn how to release your emotions)
- Remember to be aware of your vertical forehead crease when you do the exercises. Try to relax your facial expressions. Make sure your eyebrows do not knit together. Keep your face open at all times, just like your mind.

**Exercise 5: Observe Your Feelings and Your Mind**

- Observe how your emotions and thought processes affect your day. Your thoughts and feelings change your energy vibration from high to low. See how with a change of feeling and a change of thought you can easily change your perspective on a situation and feel better or worse. You are co-creating your reality at every moment. (See Chapter 5 to learn more about your Law of Attraction.)

**Exercise 6: Learn to Breathe Properly**

- Learn to breathe deeply, in and out, and loosen your facial muscles. Become conscious of your facial habits and breathing until your mind,

body, and face have been reprogrammed, and you naturally relax.
- Sit on a chair with your feet on the floor. Hold your hands palms up on your lap, just under your belly button. Relax your chest and lower your shoulders. Breathe in through your nose and out through your mouth. Breathe into your hand allowing your stomach to rise and fall naturally. Imagine you are pushing all your negative, toxic energy from your body and refilling yourself with clean, life-enhancing energy.
- Unclench your jaw, a major area for holding tension; open your eyes wide, stretch out the creases in your forehead, unfurrow your brow, allow your face to be bright and open. Imagine chewing sticky toffee to relax your mouth.
- You can also place your fingers in the center of your forehead and sweep outward in horizontal lines to release facial tension. Repeat three times.
- Now lightly press your palms onto your eye sockets and lightly sweep your fingertips down your cheek. Repeat three times.
- Any time that you sit at your computer, watch television, or read, check your breathing and the tension in your face. If you breathe deeply for five to ten minutes each day, you will begin to feel more relaxed.

**Exercise 7: Learn to Meditate**

- Close your eyes. Breathe deeply from your stomach, in and out. Allow your lips to part so your mouth relaxes. Imagine a third eye in between your eyebrows. Focus on your third eye, and then move your attention back from the third eye as if you are moving into the middle of your brain. You may see a flash of bright light appear. This means you have activated your pineal gland and opened up your second sight.
- Imagine pulling energy down through your crown chakra, down your spine to your sacrum and out through your feet. Then circle the energy back up to your crown chakra.
- Repeat this exercise circling the energy around your body. This will purify you and build a powerful energy field.

**Exercise 8: Gently Exercise Daily**

- Tai Chi or Qi Gong are gentle but powerful exercise programs to clear your energy, reduce stress, and support the body. Exercise daily with a DVD or join a class in your local community. Just thirty minutes a day will help you gain better health, fitness, and peace of mind as your mind and body work in harmony.

**Exercise 9: Foods for Healthy Facial Skin**

- Blend half an avocado with yogurt and frozen berries to make a creamy, nutty-flavored morning smoothie.
- Eat mangoes—they contain Vitamin A which maintains and repairs skin cells.
- Almonds provide 100 percent of your daily requirement for Vitamin E.
- Coconut water can cure acne scars. You can apply coconut water on your face every day.
- Cottage cheese, salmon, button mushrooms, cod, or Brazil nuts contain selenium which is an essential antioxidant mineral.
- Citrus fruits supply 100 percent of your daily allowance for Vitamin C.
- Oysters fight pimples because they are rich in zinc.
- Fruits such as apples, bananas, strawberries, tomatoes, avocados, pineapples, oranges, papayas, melons, peaches, and pears and legumes such as kidney beans, pinto beans, black-eyed peas, and lentils are rich in magnesium.
- Mushrooms are rich in riboflavin (Vitamin B2) which is involved in tissue maintenance and repair.
- Sprinkle wheat germ on yogurt for a tasty way to get more biotin in your diet.
- Eat broccoli, cauliflower, Brussels sprouts, and cabbage and add cinnamon and cardamom to your food to restore glutathione levels.
- Eat sardines, pistachios, peanuts, sesame seeds, tuna, herring, and soybeans to maintain CoQ10 levels.

**Exercise 10: Nourish the Brain and Take a Natural Anti-Wrinkle Supplement**

- Take a high grade Vitamin B-Complex and a daily liquid trace mineral formula (especially chromium) to nourish the brain.
- Take gingko to improve memory loss.
- Also feed the brain omega fatty acids. Take a tablespoon of fish oil or

flaxseed oil every day or add flaxseed meal to your smoothie, yogurt, salad, cereals, or oatmeal. This will make deeply etched wrinkles disappear and keep acne at bay.

- Take a zinc and magnesium supplement to maintain hyaluronic acid levels, collagen, and elastin fibers that preserve skin's elasticity and firmness.
- Take Vitamin C to fight skin damage, prevent wrinkles, and maintain collagen.
- Take a glutathione and CoQ10 supplement as a powerful antioxidant.
- Minimize cell phone use.

**Exercise 11: Bathe in Magnesium**

- Bathe in an Epsom salts bath three times a week.
- You can also use magnesium oil as an alternative to Epsom salts.

**Exercise 12: Herbal Relief for the Mind**

- Passionflower is considered a mild sedative and can help promote sleep. Passionflower also treats anxiety, depression, and nervousness.
- St. John's Wort has been used medicinally since Hippocrates' time. Even during the Renaissance and Victorian periods, it was used for the treatment of mental disorders. St. John's Wort has been shown to be more effective than Prozac.
- Lavender is effective at reducing irritability and anxiety, promoting relaxation, a sense of calm, and sleep. While lavender can be consumed in a tea, it works best as an essential oil that is breathed in by way of a diffuser or in the case of stress and sleeplessness, an eye pillow.

**Exercise 13: Aromatherapy for Depression**

- People who suffer from depression may benefit from aromatherapy. The sense of smell is closely associated with emotional centers in the brain. Essential oils stimulate both the endocrine system and the limbic area of the brain—each one is a key component in the prevention of depression.
- Essential oils may be used in diffusion (essential oil drops in water for inhalation) or with a body massage. In aromatherapy, the following

essential oils are generally regarded as being uplifting and helpful in depression: bergamot, chamomile, jasmine, sandalwood, geranium, rose, or peppermint.

- Book a session with a highly qualified aromatherapist or ask your partner to massage you with essential oils.

### Exercise 14: Oxygenation and Skin Color

Follow these exercises to oxygenate your skin and heighten your skin tone.

- Find the apple of your cheeks and press your index finger there. This will detoxify and oxygenate the skin.
- This is an ancient Indian facial yoga technique that brings circulation to the face. Pull your middle earlobes out to the sides with your thumb and index finger four times. Grab your lower earlobes and pull down lightly four times. Then grab your upper earlobes and pull up four times. This will heighten your skin color.
- To ensure proper blood and oxygen circulation around your brain, bend over and massage your head for five minutes a day. You can also book a cranium sacral massage to release any pressure points in your skull.

### Exercise 15: Cleanse and Moisturize

- Cleanse your face twice daily. Use gentle and safe skin care products—organic whenever possible. At night, make sure you remove your makeup and cleanse properly before you go to bed. Use an oil-free makeup remover. It is very damaging for your skin to get into bed leaving makeup and environmental grime on your face while you sleep.
- Once your face is clean, moisturize with a good, natural face cream that is oil free. Ideally, your face cream should contain alpha lipoeic acids, alpha hydroxy acids, amino acids, Vitamin A, C, and E, peptides and peptide complexes or hyaluronic acid or CoQ10. You can also use an organic face cream containing beeswax or zinc oxide to renew collagen.
- Apply your skin care products gently to warm skin. The warmth maximizes absorption. Lightly tap your skin for a few moments to help it absorb them.

- Do not rub or pull your face. Rubbing stretches your skin and can promote sagging and wrinkles.
- Remember to sleep on your back instead of your front so you minimize creasing your face. If you press your face to your pillow, you will experience increased puffiness in the morning.
- Use at least a thirty factor sunscreen with only natural ingredients.
- During the winter months you can use Vaseline cream if you are going out for a walk. This age old remedy will give you an extra layer of protection and will stop your skin from chaffing. Petroleum jelly can also be used as a temporary lip balm, hand, and feet moisturizer. You can find a nonpetroleum multi-purpose jelly with natural ingredients from natural beauty companies such as Alba. This cream can be used to prevent dryness, chaffing, and windburn and is also great for removing eye makeup.

## Exercise 16: Nightly Facial Massage

- Give yourself a facial massage whenever you are watching television or have a resting moment in your day. Work your fingers through the skin of your forehead to smooth away the deep crevices and wrinkles. Use your index fingers or your knuckles to mold deeply the skin upwards and out with circular motions. A great acupressure point lies between your nose and your eyes. Press your index fingers or thumbs under the inner arch of your eyebrows. Tap the ridge above your eyebrows. This is also helpful for smoothing facial lines and preventing wrinkles
- Use natural oils such as Vitamin E or coconut oil with your nightly massage so you do not "burn" the skin.

## Exercise 17: Weekly Exfoliation

- Use a gentle exfoliator such as ground oatmeal, barley, or a ground almond and yogurt scrub. Once a week you may want to make a face mask of avocado and sesame oil. Leave it on for half an hour; then rinse your face with warm water and pat it dry.
- Or take one tablespoon of whipped egg white and a squeeze of lemon. Smooth it over your face, avoiding the eye area, and wash off after ten minutes.

- Or add five teaspoons of baking soda to approximately two tablespoons of a gentle facial cleanser or two tablespoons of purified water. Mix thoroughly. The goal is to create a thick paste. If you have sensitive skin, use less baking soda. Add a little of the paste to your premoistened face, starting on your forehead. Massage lightly into the skin with a damp washcloth using circular motions. Add more paste as needed. Rinse off with tepid water. Gently pat dry. Limit exfoliation to twice per week.
- Make a cup of green tea and leave enough in your cup to make a green tea face mask. Green tea has many benefits externally as well as internally. As a skin calmer and healer, it is gentle enough to use on the most sensitive of skin. You can also add honey and porridge oats to make a green tea paste.
- Add cucumber to any of the above facial masks to improve complexion or cucumber can also be used as a toner to tighten pores. Blend cucumber with apple cider vinegar or lemon juice, egg white, honey, or aloe. Cucumber skin is especially beneficial.

**Exercise 18: Mineral Makeup**

- There are harmful chemicals found in most makeup products so switch to high quality mineral cosmetics if you want to protect and preserve your skin.

**Exercise 19: Crystals for Calming the Mind and Erasing Wrinkles**

- For mental health, balance, and healing carry alexandrite, celestite, sugilite, or tourmaline crystals. Place the crystal on your third eye for thirty minutes.
- Drinking a pink opal elixir can be calming and comforting for all types of mental unrest.
- To help release wrinkles, carry or wear aragonite, rose quartz, or selenite. You can also drink a lipidolite elixir.
- For skin elasticity, carry or wear selenite or apply gypsum elixir to your skin.
- For acne, carry or wear amethyst, amber, jade, or selenite or even place a larger crystal by your bed. Place any of the crystals on your worst

spot. You can also make an overnight amber elixir, and apply it to your skin.

- For a youthful appearance, add rose quartz to your bath or carry and wear moonstone, sapphire, selenite, or sodalite.
- For the vertical crease on your forehead, hold, wear, or carry wulfenite which helps you see, face, and deal with your dark side.

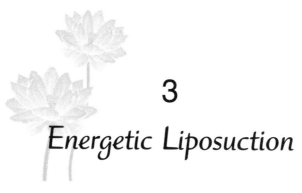

# 3

# Energetic Liposuction

*Man shall not live by bread alone*
*but by every word that proceedeth out of the mouth of God.*
**Jesus Christ**

Weight issues, excess cellulite, and body fat are an ongoing problem for many people. They walk around with low self-esteem and deep depression because no matter how much they change their diet, they still seem to be heavier than their ideal weight. If you are one such person, then I am here to tell you that there is hope; you can create the body that God intended for you. The perpetual cycle of dieting can end and not through stapling your body or dangerous liposuction procedures.

But to lose weight, you do not need just a change of diet but a whole new mindset. You have to look at your body fat in an entirely new way. Remember that your body is not just solid matter made up of flesh, blood, and bone–it is energy materialized into matter. I have heard many stories about highly trained yogis in the East, who can materialize and dematerialize their physical body in front of people. They can gain or lose ten pounds overnight. They are able to do this because they understand their bodies are made of energy, and they have learned to change their energy field from a low frequency to a higher frequency vibration. The faster the body vibrates, the more it disappears–a little like a fan spinning so quickly that you do not see the individual blades anymore.

When you change your relationship and your perception of your body and start to embrace the fact that your body is made of energy rather than focus on the solid image reflected back at you in the mirror, you then will begin to understand how to control your weight and change your body shape.

## What Is Weight?

In Chapter 1 you learned about energy frequencies running through your body and that you have a soul, a spirit body, and a physical body. You also learned about your soul condition and how the energy in your soul, your spirit body, and your physical body can affect the way you look, feel, and age. You also learned in Chapter 2 how your thoughts and internal reactions to external events create your facial wrinkles and how these thoughts originate from the negative feelings in your soul. You can now start to move ahead with losing weight and dealing with these feelings. You can finally clear the dense, heavy energy that has collected in your cells over the years. But first, let us understand how your weight got there in the first place.

Your weight is determined by your soul condition, or more importantly, what is contained in your soul. Remember that your soul is made up of your passions, desires, emotions, aspirations, intentions, free will, memories, personality, instincts, and natural love, but it is your emotions that are the seat of your soul and you have absorbed a whole array of them since childhood. Those emotions that are in harmony with love make you feel happy and loving towards yourself and others. They keep your energy field light, purified, and vibrating quickly, which helps your body and chakra system function properly. But unfortunately, more often than not, the contents of our souls are out of harmony with love. The negative emotions we carry are heavy and energetically dense. They cause us pain due to an error–based upbringing and environmental belief systems.

Think of your emotions as *energy in motion* (e–motion.) Every emotion is a substance that is transmitted and changes the substance of your soul and your physical body. The *e-motion-al* injuries enter your cells from your soul via your spirit body or aura and change into solid matter in your physical body. If negative emotions are inhibited, then the energy of that emotion becomes stuck, creating a physical imbalance. This blocks the flow of energy through your chakra system and disrupts how your body functions. Remember, just like everything else in the universe, all your emotions have an electromagnetic charge. Negative emotions, especially, have a strong emotional charge that can drain the aura.

The unhealthy energy changes the energy of your cells to a slow, dense frequency that begins to age you and causes you to put on weight. Positive, loving, high–frequency emotions also have an emotional charge, but they flow quickly and smoothly; they boost the energy supply and affect the body in a healthy way.

When you were conceived, your soul was in pristine condition without emotional injuries, but it automatically began to absorb emotions from its environment. That means that as soon as you were conceived, you started absorbing all the energy of your mother's suppressed feelings when you were inside her womb. Most probably, many of these suppressed emotions were toxic and out of harmony with love. Then you started to absorb your father's suppressed emotions after you were born. This absorption of your parents' suppressed emotions changed your soul condition, filled your container with negativity, and changed your body's energy field, causing you great harm. This contamination continued until you were grown up.

In a normal state a child always feels its own as well as environmental emotions. If an adult suppresses his or her emotion, then the child is forced to feel the adult's emotion as well. Many parents are unaware how much they are harming their children due to their actions and emotional suppression. They want to love their children, but they do not know how to love properly. This is due to their emotional injuries, learned societal and ancestral belief systems, and a lack of understanding about God's laws.

Your parents most probably curtailed your free will so they could control you even though the Law of Free Will is one of the most important laws God ever gifted to humans. As a child with a lack of free will and living in your parents' home, you had no escape from absorbing your protectors' suppressed emotions or being on the end of their unloving, controlling actions, such as shouting, hitting, or denying you

## Our Emotions Reflect Those of Our Parents and Our Environment

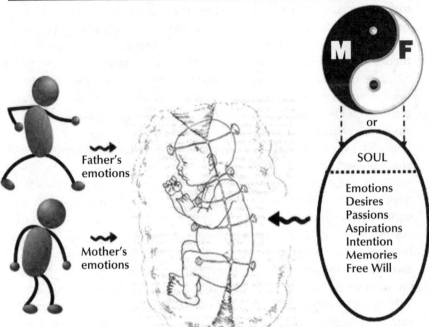

Father's
emotions

Mother's
emotions

or

SOUL

Emotions
Desires
Passions
Aspirations
Intention
Memories
Free Will

Emotions flow to unborn baby, then from those around the baby when it is born.

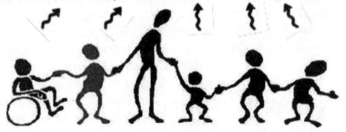

The soul half that incarnates is the one most suitable for the characteristics of the attracting parents. Upon incarnation, the soul's condition adjusts to reflect the soul condition of the parents. Children absorb and reflect the emotions of their parents, their ancestors, and those around them, such as teachers, neighbors, and grandparents. If these emotions are negative and get blocked or frozen in the soul, they cause harm to the body.

your feelings. Unable to know what to do with the bombardment of toxic emotions you had to deal with, you started to create your own negative emotions as a reaction. Instead of honoring your free will and allowing you to naturally process your negative emotions, your parents then suppressed you further to avoid their own emotions.

Emotions that are not completely experienced get stored (frozen) in the soul. They are only released from the soul when they are completely experienced. It is the emotional charge that holds the pattern in storage until it is consciously activated and released.

When a child is prevented from feeling an emotion, the emotion gets stuck. The child then responds in rage or anger because his or her free will is not being allowed. These reactions attract a chain of other reactions and events in his or her life that are also out of harmony with love, such as spanking. These abusive occurrences result in the child's soul becoming more and more contaminated with toxic emotions that cause him or her severe emotional pain and bodily harm. The further we move away from core emotions, the further we are from our true selves. We are designed to feel emotions because emotions are the seat of the soul.

It was not only your parents that harmed you as you were growing up, because grandparents, family friends, and teachers at school also surrounded you. All of these adults were carrying suppressed emotional wounds from their childhoods, and many of their emotions and actions towards you were out of harmony with love. These actions also caused you emotional harm whether or not the adults were aware of what they were doing and deliberately meant to hurt you.

## RELEASING THE FAMILY BLUEPRINT

As you read in Chapter 1, the vibrations of our thoughts, beliefs, and emotions become embedded and carried in our DNA from generation to generation. Many dysfunctional behavioral patterns and negative emotions get stored in the cells and passed down through the ancestral line. The emotional blueprint of a family is strong and powerful; nearly every generation stays loyal to it. The blueprint goes back as far as four generations. This is all very well if the family traditions, beliefs, and behaviors are in harmony with love, but most of the time they are harmful and completely disharmonious. Spanking, for instance, goes completely against God's laws of Natural Love. The root of this practice may be found in these examples. Perhaps your family is African American, and you were once slaves and were beaten by your white owners. It might be that your parents were sent to boarding school and received corporal punishment so the whipping and beating of children has been accepted as a form of discipline in your family and passed down through the ancestral line.

It is very common for the abused to become the abuser and pass on emotional, mental, or physical violence from generation to generation. But any form of abuse against another is unloving, especially if it is an adult trying to physically punish a child. It breaks God's laws of Natural Love and instills an emotional penalty on the soul, which degrades the soul's condition and therefore, the physical body.

There are many more examples of family codes and blueprints that are passed down the family line which harm the next generation. Perhaps you come from a family that lives in a culture which focuses on intellectual development rather than emotional expression. Your family may have an obsession with the accumulation of material wealth rather than emphasizing spiritual progression. It could be that a great-grandmother was raped, and her hatred of men was passed down through the female members of the family line. It might also be that your grandfather was involved in Hiroshima or the Holocaust, and his experience of loss and suppressed grief has been repeated in your own life. These different ancestral patterns damage a child's soul. The family blueprint then becomes ingrained in the cells of every generation. Emotional memories and cellular damage gets passed down from great grandparents, grandparents, and parents to their children.

If you research the stories of your ancestors, you will find many similar belief systems, behavioral patterns, illnesses, addictions, everyday problems, and emotional injuries that affect you and your family today. It is this emotional family blueprint that you need to clear from your body, mind, and soul if you want to return to your natural state. When you crack the code and clear the cellular damage, your cells will alter. You will no longer remember the negative past event nor will your cells. Your body will heal from unhealthy generational belief systems, abuse, and past traumas, and your DNA will change.

But breaking the family blueprint can be incredibly hard for people to do because they feel guilty and duty-bound to stay loyal to family traditions. It can take time to break through the code that binds you, but do not give up trying to release it. If you are emotionally honest, you can access the pattern you need to release. If you do not break the family blueprint, then you will never get to know your own soul, fulfill your own soul's purpose, or reach a state of perfected love. You will end up living in someone else's painful past and not in the joy of your present life.

## WHAT FEELINGS ARE YOU EATING?

Even though our emotions are the seat of our soul, are the most vital guide on our journey through life, and their release is of the utmost importance for our health and well-being, most people have been taught to suppress the way they feel due to the stigma that exists in society about discussing feelings, especially negative ones. People are too ashamed to be emotionally honest. They were shut down from feeling their real emotions when they were young and have never been given the tools to release emotions so as an adult they carry an array of harmful feelings inside of them such as anger, grief, resentment, shame, and fear.

### Examples of Harmful Emotions

| | | | | |
|---|---|---|---|---|
| Anger | Frustration | Hate | Fear | Jealousy |
| Shame | Irritation | Guilt | Malice | Unworthiness |
| Hurt | Dejection | Despair | Regret | Helplessness |
| Disgust | Outrage | Hostility | Coldness | Indignant |
| Stressed | Exhausted | Numb | Bored | Loneliness |
| Guarded | Hopelessness | Sensitive | Alarmed | Self-Consciousness |

Because these emotions become stored or frozen in the soul and the flow of feelings gets blocked, the e-motion becomes motionless and the energy gets stuck. It builds up and becomes dense. This dense emotion starts to weigh you down, leading to excess body fat. Furthermore, emotional blocks are held in your tissue, causing the connective tissue to alter its structure. The tissue then buries itself in your body and changes into cellulite. The longer the emotions remain unresolved in your body, the more severe the effect. Your body does not just gain weight but becomes imbalanced. Every negative emotion that is stored in your soul makes you more susceptible to disease and death.

Even though many people know that negative emotions are harmful, they would rather push their emotions down inside than deal with the pain of feeling them, but your body does not want to deal with them any more than you do. Unless you can free your body of these blockages, these emotional congestions are like lethal hand grenades within your physical body that are ready to go off at any minute. They not only cause you illness but also negatively affect your Law of Attraction. Remember, the electromagnetic charge of your emotion attracts electromagnetically charged energy from your environment that is of a similar frequency. Your stored negative emotions create all sorts of negative events in your life that cause further pain, illness, and obesity. (See Chapter 5.)

Despite these known hazards, both men and women have been taught to suppress their negative feelings. Men have been taught not to cry; they learn to remain emotionally stoic and strong. Their suppressed grief gets turned into outbursts of aggression and anger. Even though it is acceptable for a woman to cry, she has been taught to feel ashamed of admitting her darker feelings, such as rage or anger. An angry woman is seen as unladylike. She has been taught to appease and be the good girl. Both men and women have overcompensated for their emotional suppression by staying focused on making the physical body and intellectual mind more visually perfect and powerful.

Women, especially, have obsessed over perfecting their looks; they smile and look pretty when deep down inside they feel vengeful and angry. This denial of emotions has caused many people to function from their upper chakras. Most women are cut off at the waist, living from the top half of their bodies. Not only are they are disconnected from their souls, the containers for their emotions, but also from their wombs, which store their deeper emotions in their physical bodies. This "out of body" existence and deep disconnect helps them to tune out of life and to avoid experiencing their painful feelings. Going out of body often happens when someone has gone through a traumatic event. Any time people feel threatened, their need to guard or defend usually results in holding the breath or breathing in shallow, erratic patterns. When they gasp with the shock of the event, they take a sharp in breath, lift up and out of their bodies, and there they stay forever more. For the rest of their lives their bodies are tense, and they breathe only from their chest rather than from their stomach. They remain deeply traumatized by what has happened to them but are now numb to their real feelings.

Unfortunately, as they walk through life, emotionally disconnected and traumatized, their cells still retain the trauma, their body gets heavier and their hips wider. They fill up with the dense energy of suppressed resentment, guilt, fear, grief, shame and anger. This emotional suppression causes diseases such as breast cancer. My motto to all women is: "Get your feelings off your chest, not your breasts." I firmly believe that breast cancer is caused by suppressed grief and anger and a desire to over nurture others more than you because of a need to be loved. Likewise, throat cancer is also caused by an inability to speak your emotional truth. As you fail to express your deepest, darkest feelings, the throat chakra gets blocked. The second chakra also becomes blocked with negative emotions which can lead to uterine cancer. Remember, you can find the root cause of all of the issues creating your ill health by looking at the role and function of the correlating chakra (see chapter 1).

All disease stems from trauma (i.e. a sudden loss or accident), an emotional injury relating back to the father or the mother, and from a weakness in the cells of your body passed down through the generations of your family line. The deep cellular wounds and emotional charge of the memories of the past block the flow of energy through your chakra system. The negative emotions also create an acidic reaction in the water of the cells of your body, which causes your cells to mutate. If your PH level is out of balance, then disease occurs. You will read more about the causes and effects of an acidic body in Chapter 5. The only way to release the deep trauma and toxic emotions that cause illness and heavy weight is to climb back down into the body. From this place of renewed connection, all people can start breathing and feeling again so that their bodies and their souls can heal.

## WHAT ARE YOU DOING TO NUMB YOURSELF?

Because of the stigma about speaking about our inner most feelings, people try to avoid their pain by anesthetizing themselves with numbing agents such as television, food, alcohol, cigarettes, shopping, drugs, sex, or prescription medications. Even coffee is an antidepressant used to avoid emotions. By the time most people get to their twenties, thirties, forties, and upwards, they are carrying around so many toxic layers of pain because of these physical addictions that they have doubled in size, overwhelmed their systems, and become emotionally numb.

Even many Eastern gurus, New Thought teachers, and self–help motivators encourage a detunement or a disconnect from emotions. The motto to their followers is: "Change your mind and change your life." Meditation is also used by some people to "zen out of life," just as the addict does with food, alcohol, or drugs. Meditation can make an emotional avoider feel temporarily high and can numb him or her from feeling. I explained in Chapter 2 that meditation should be a supportive tool and not become an addiction or a replacement for emotional processing. Your thoughts come from your feelings, and the mind is not the soul. The only way for you to become purified and free from suffering is never to ignore the emotion that you feel. That is who you are at the moment. If you tell yourself the story that you want to be something different and try to change your mind, then you are forcing yourself away from your true emotional condition. You have to recognize the truth of the moment and the truth of your feelings. Your feelings are your guide, and ignoring them is dangerous.

When you numb yourself and detune from your own emotions, you not only disconnect from your soul, your true self, but also from other people. This creates a feeling of isolation and even more pain. The end result is that the pain becomes so unbearable and the void so intense that you reach for something to fill you up and comfort you; more often than not this something is food—usually the junk kind. Now your body is not only full of toxic feelings but also toxic food. The food creates short-term comfort but also adds more layers on top of the layers of pain. The layers help you feel like your inner child is being protected, similar to wearing several jackets when you go out into the cold. The food and the suppressed emotions replace the comfort blanket you carried around when you were young. Chapter 5 will discuss further the importance of understanding the energy frequencies of different foods and how they affect body weight, our internal organs, and outer skin, but for now we will continue to focus on processing your toxic emotions.

## ACCESSING CAUSAL EMOTIONS

Hopefully you now understand how you gained your weight and how important it is to release your negative emotions as soon as they enter. You do not want to let emotions fester in your body and create more weight and health problems. But how do you reverse the damage that you have already done to your body? How do you release your emotional toxins, make your body "lighter," permanently give up dieting, and become your perfect weight? The only way to lose your weight permanently is to peel the pain layers away. You have to take your bundle of protective jackets off and strip yourself emotionally bare. You do this by learning to feel your *causal emotions*. It is only by experiencing and expressing causal emotions that you can release them. Experiencing an emotion releases the block. No one else can feel your emotions and do this for you.

But what are causal emotions? A causal emotion is the original emotion that was the cause of your pain. It is the negative feeling that you had when you were a child that has created a series of events and emotions in your life ever since. Your causal emotion generates your Law of Attraction. What you feel and what you think about, you create. That means that whatever is happening in your life at this present time is due to the causal emotions in your soul.

If you are perfectly happy, you attract only abundance, love, and good things into your life. If you are never upset, frightened, guilty, irritated, or angry, that means you do not have negative causal emotions in your soul. But if you attract people that annoy you or if you experience conflict in your work, family, or romantic life, that means you are being negatively affected by causal emotions in your soul. Remember that childhood causal emotional damage is created by people in a child's environment who are suppressing their own emotional experiences. Because you have been forced to suppress yourself since you were a child, you can imagine that you have a lot of causal emotions stored deep down inside.

Below is a discussion of the four types of causal emotions that you have absorbed and carried inside of you since you were young: *how others have hurt others, how others have hurt you, how you have hurt yourself,* and *how you have hurt others.* Once you have accessed your causal emotions, you can start to release them and change your weight and your life.

## 1. How Others Have Hurt Others

From the moment you were born, you watched as others around you have hurt each other. You may have seen your parents shout, or worse still, hit and abuse each other. They may have thrown a hurtful, sarcastic comment across the dinner table. Even if your childhood home was a perfect sanctuary of love, as soon as your parents turned on the television set, you saw murders, animal cruelty, child abuse, and wars flashing across the screen. These destructive, unloving images seared into your heart and soul and flooded the living room with toxic energy that you, then, absorbed. If people do not release the hurt they absorb from the external events they witness, then every painful emotion gets stuck or frozen in their souls. They get weighed down with emotions as they see a homeless person being stepped over in the street, the elderly being deserted by family members, parents hitting a child, starving people dying, or an innocent animal harmed by the hand of a cruel human. If you are to clear your soul, lose weight, and reshape your body, you need to purge your emotions of *how others have hurt others.*

## 2. How Others Have Hurt You

As I have already written, many parents are unloving not because they are bad people, but because they are damaged and do not know how to love properly. Even if you had a happy childhood, there were moments when your needs were not met in some way or other. You, therefore, need to purge your stored childhood emotions from your cellular body. It is important that you remove negative emotions caused by both of your parents. It affects everything else that is happening in your life, since 80 percent of how we learn to love comes from our mother and 80 percent of our self-esteem comes from our father.

It can be hard to face the truth about our parents. If you are a man, then it can be especially hard to face the facts about your father because he is the same sex as you; the same applies to women and their mothers. It is easier to feel the emotional injuries caused by a parent of the opposite sex. There is also a big taboo about the mother—as the saying goes: "Mother knows best." It is hard to find a song about a woman or bad mother but quite a few songs are written about a man or a father. But I promise you that there have been times in your life when your mother, because of her emotional injuries, was just as unloving to you as your father was. You have probably spent 80 percent of your childhood with your mother while your father was working, so she has had more of an effect on the condition of your soul than anyone else in your family. The role of the mother and how she impacts our ability to love is further discussed in Chapter 4.

Once you have released your feelings about your parents, then you will have to purge how other adults, family members, teachers, or family friends have hurt you. You have to release the family blueprint and the feelings of guilt that you may feel when you do so. Finally, you will have to access the negative emotions frozen in your soul that have been caused by your environment, the false societal beliefs or systems, such as racism and sexism, or the oppressive political regimes and religious institutions that are out of harmony with God's laws. You have been hurt many times in your lifetime so if you are to lose weight, it is important that you release all your emotions about *how others have hurt you.*

## 3. How You Have Hurt Yourself

When children have been hurt or emotionally repressed, they will often harm themselves as a reaction. They feel unlovable or angry and frustrated so they do unloving actions to themselves because they have not been given emotional tools to cope.

This self-abuse and self-destruction can often be carried into adulthood. As adults, they put themselves in harm's way, eat unhealthily, take drugs and alcohol, enter into abusive relationships, become sexually promiscuous, deny themselves their passions and desires, push away those that love them, end up living to only half their potentials, or give their power away and undervalue themselves. If you are to lose weight, you have to purge all of the emotions that have accumulated in your lifetime because of *how you have hurt yourself.*

## 4. How You Have Hurt Others

The emotions of how we have hurt others are often the hardest to access. This is because we prefer to blame someone else instead of looking at our part in hurting another human. Often we are oblivious to how we have hurt others because we are so disconnected and numb to our own emotions that we are unable to be empathetic or compassionate to another's feelings. There are many things you have done in your lifetime that have hurt others—whether that be a harsh word, a thoughtless action, or a deliberate act of malice. Some of the things we do on a daily basis harm others, such as eating meat. We get someone else to kill the animals we eat so we can avoid our emotions around killing another. The animal comes nicely packaged so it is unrecognizable. I am not telling you whether or not you should eat meat, that is your own free will and choice (although a vegetarian diet will help you lose weight!) but what emotions do you feel when I tell you to get a knife and slit the throat of the animal you are about to eat? Some people do not mind killing an animal with their bare hands, but for most of us the thought of that is unbearable. That is the emotion you need to process out of your soul. The emotion of killing animals is in there whether or not you want to feel it.

The emotions that have accumulated in your soul by your unloving behaviors towards others are affecting your cells today. If you want to purify your body and lose weight, then you will have to turn your eyes inwards instead of looking outside yourself and blaming someone else. You need to finally take full emotional responsibility and purge your soul of *how you have hurt others.*

## CLEARING CAUSAL EMOTIONS

God created us to experience every one of our emotions. One important quote in the Bible is: "I tell you the truth, unless you change and become like little children, you will never enter the Kingdom of Heaven." (Matthew: 18:3) We should take note of this quote. It means that not only should we love with an open, unconditional heart like a child, but we should also process our feelings like children if we are to stay pure and reach a state of perfected love—a heavenly place inside of ourselves. If you watch children, they will cry on the spot when they are upset. They do not observe themselves and say, "Oh, I'm upset; I'd better not cry. I'll eat a piece of chocolate instead or avoid my feelings by doing something else." No, children process their emotions right then and there if they are allowed to. They have a good cry, and once they have finished releasing their grief, hurt, anger, or fear, the emotion is cleared from their souls, and they continue on with their day. This process of instantaneous, shame-free emotional processing keeps them happy, healthy, and energetically purified.

But when you were born, you were most probably told not to cry. "Hush, hush, my child, it's alright; don't cry" or "Don't be a baby. Stop crying." Adults around you probably told you to stop crying either with words or a slap on the leg. They shut you down from expressing your true feelings so that they could control you or because they did not want to feel their own suppressed emotions. This caused you terrible damage because your suppressed emotions got frozen in your soul.

If you are ever going to lose your weight permanently, you need to learn to be childlike again and shamelessly *feel* and *release* all of your emotions. You have to climb back into your body as you learn to grieve and feel again. You have to reunite your upper chakra system with your lower chakra system so the energy can flow properly, and if you are a woman reading this book, you have to reconnect with your womb—your feeling center. From this place deep down you can start to clear all of your festering emotions and trauma.

This childlike feel–and–release process begins firstly by accessing and experiencing all the causal emotions that are frozen in your soul. Remember that to experience the emotion is to release it. Emotional processing starts with being humble. The true meaning of humility is to have a passionate desire to feel all your emotions all of the time. This starts by being emotionally honest. Children are emotionally humble. They have a desire to honestly feel all of their emotions all of the time. This is why the saying "the truth will set you free" is correct because when you experience the truth and you are emotionally honest, you release the blocks and free yourself from suffering.

People try to avoid the truth at all costs because they believe the truth is too painful. But remember that it is not the truth entering you that is causing you pain, it is the error leaving your soul and the painful emotional injuries clearing from your body when you hear the truth that is hurting you. When you connect with truth and feel your pain, you allow the error to leave. The more you connect to the truth by speaking it out loud, the more you can feel and release your causal emotions and clear the emotional injuries. If you stay emotionally honest, this "truth–feel–release" experience will help you remove all the emotional errors from your soul.

"But, I hear you cry; I can't bear to feel the pain. It makes me feel worse than I already feel." I promise you that feeling and releasing your emotions are the greatest gifts you can give to yourself, even if it causes you some intense pain for a short while. Emotions attached to your past experiences probably have a strong charge; the likelihood of them being trapped in your body is very high. Unless you delve into the experiences of your past and release your stored negative emotions, you are headed into an emotionally, mentally, spiritually, and physically painful life.

Imagine walking around with a thorn in your shoe every day, and even though you take the shoe off to ease the pain every night and it makes you feel better for a while, the wound in your foot is still there. It opens up again the very next day when you put the shoe back on. It just gets deeper and harder to heal; you are in even more pain for the rest of the day. It is better to take the thorn out once and for all, even if it hurts intensely for a while. Once the wound has healed, you will never have to deal with the recurring pain again. This is what you need to do with the wounds in your soul. You need to pierce through your blocks and access your suppressed emotions. Trust the saying: "Short-term pain for long-term gain."

Perhaps reminding you about your Law of Attraction will give you another incentive. Remember that when you release the emotion completely, your Law of Attraction changes. If you do not release the negative emotions, their electromagnetic charge will continue to attract negative events. So if you want to stop painful things from happening in your life, breathe in deeply from your stomach, speak the emotional truth out loud, feel your emotions, and release them even if that truth is: "My mother did not love me" or "My father did not value me." "My partner is abusive, and I do not love him anymore." Start from that painful truth and let your grief pour out. Release your grief, have a good cry so that suppressed emotions no longer control your weight or the events in your life. Once the emotional injury and causal emotion are cleared from your soul, you will never have to feel them again. It will not attract in a negative event. You will feel no emotional charge when you speak about a person or event. You will know your soul is totally clear from the injury when you have no tears and feel no pain. Then your Law of Attraction changes and brings you only peaceful or happy things.

As the causal emotion releases, so your body will purge the dense energy and change. This feel-and-release process is great for reducing bulging stomachs and thighs. Your body will get lighter as the negative emotions are removed. If you make this feel-and-release process part of your daily routine, you will soon learn to feel an emotion without feeling good or bad about it. This does not mean you are blocking the emotion but simply feeling it, experiencing and releasing it without any judgment, just as you did all those years ago when you were a child.

## IDENTIFYING CAPPING EMOTIONS

Now that you know how to access and release your causal emotions, you are well on your way to losing weight. But quite often accessing your grief or the emotions that cause your pain can be difficult because you are focused on another emotion other than your actual causal emotion. This other emotion can block as well as confuse you and stop you from accessing your true feelings. This is called a *blocking or capping emotion.*

Imagine that you are a child and you accidently knock over a vase in your parents' home. Instead of your mother reassuring you that it is okay and that everyone makes mistakes, she yanks you away and yells at you. You start to cry, but she continues to shout about her best vase and calls you stupid. She sends you to your room and threatens that your father will spank you when he gets home. The cause of your emotion (the causal emotion) is the fact that your mother is being unloving to you and is now contaminating your soul. You are crying because an emotional error from your mother has entered you. You now feel unworthy, unlovable, and stupid. You need to grieve and release these emotions. But your grieving process is interrupted by the extra emotion of feeling frightened of being punished by your father. Then your father comes home and spanks you, which makes you very angry.

The causal emotion (the grief of having an unloving mother and feeling stupid and unworthy) is now superceded by other emotions of fear and anger. These are called *capping emotions.* Capping emotions cover up the actual cause of your pain. They cover up your causal emotions.

In the space of a few hours your perfect world has been shattered along with the vase. You have learned that you are stupid, that your mother controls your father's actions, and that neither your mother nor your father are unconditionally loving or forgiving; they are most certainly not your protectors. You have a lot of emotions of grief to process underneath the surface, but you no longer feel your grief because your capping emotion has taken over. The once innocent, loving you is now angry. You become unloving to other people in your words and actions because you are angry and denying your actual causal emotions.

People operate from their capping emotions as they grow up, completely blocked from their original grief and causal emotion. A capping emotion sits on top of the causal emotion and creates another layer of pain. Grief is the causal emotion and then on top of grief is fear (the fear of feeling the grief.) Rage and hatred sit on top of the fear, and after anger we go numb. When we become numb, we suffer from depression. People numb themselves because they are ashamed of their anger and fearful of any type of emotional pain; they do not want to feel their causal emotions. When people are numb, they detune from their own pain. They become depressed, take antidepressants that have side effects, and fill up their days to avoid their true feelings. If they could just move beyond their fear to the actual causal emotion and allow that emotion to come up and out of them, then they would overcome their depression and start to feel alive again. Many times people do not even realize the original causal emotion is still there beneath all of their fear, rage, and eventual numbness.

If you feel overwhelmed after reading this section about capping emotions because you see how many different layers of pain have accumulated over the years that you have to remove, please take a deep breath. We have always been taught that when we are overwhelmed, we cannot cope, but we can cope if we emotionally process. Yes, it is true; you have many emotional injuries inside you that have caused your weight gain, but these wounds can easily be accessed if you are willing to feel your causal emotions. The rest of your capping emotions will dissolve away when you get right to the core of your pain and remove the original causal emotion. Just work your way through your causal emotions, and you will begin to see the light of day and the lighter weight of your body.

## WHAT ARE EMOTIONS OF SELF-DECEPTION?

Rage and anger are common reactions for most people. These are known as *emotions of self-deception*. When we deny our own emotional experience, we project the emotion outwards and get angry. Anger is emotional dishonesty—an inability to be emotionally humble. We get stuck in anger or blame to avoid our own feelings. We are frightened to feel our causal emotion in case it is too painful, but we do not want to admit that we are frightened so we express anger instead. When we are angry, it makes us feel powerful and in control; we project our feelings onto someone else because we do not want to feel our own pain. Because we grow up being told we cannot feel our emotions, we try to get other people to feel them instead when we become adults. As long as you stay in anger and blame, you will deny your grief, and the negative emotions will fester and damage your body. When you take responsibility for your own emotions, then you will not get angry with another person.

If there are two lessons that I hope you take away from reading this book, it is these: when you are angry, you are avoiding your causal emotions, and no one can feel your feelings for you; only *you* can feel and release your own emotions. Anger, irritation, rage, blame, and

## We Need to Feel Capping Emotions

We are made to feel emotions. We shut down our emotions instead of nurturing and processing them. We blame ourselves or blame others. We need to feel our capping and causal emotions. The further away from causal emotions, the further we are away from our true selves.

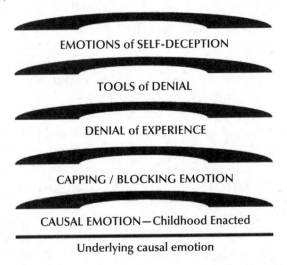

EMOTIONS of SELF-DECEPTION

TOOLS of DENIAL

DENIAL of EXPERIENCE

CAPPING / BLOCKING EMOTION

CAUSAL EMOTION—Childhood Enacted

Underlying causal emotion

Children reflect their parents' suppressed emotions. The parents' anger is a reflection of their emotional denial. The underlying causal emotion reflects the causal event. Move through the anger into the grief.

depression are all examples of the emotions of self-deception.

If you play the blame game, you will never heal your life. When you project your feelings on someone else, your Law of Attraction will be affected and will never change. You will have more painful events and physical complaints enter your life because you are not releasing the causal emotion that created the event in the first place. If you do not come to terms with this truth, then you will always be angry with someone else. Your anger will harm your body and potentially kill you.

Do not feel guilty if you have anger come up inside of you; do not add to your feelings of unworthiness and self-loathing. Just as it is important not to blame or get angry at another person, do not fall into the trap of blaming and punishing yourself either. Blame and self-punishment are a waste of time and energy. Self-blame helps you only to avoid your causal emotion. If you did do something wrong, then connect to your grief about what you have lost in your life and connect to the causal emotion that made you do something harmful in the first place. The reason that events and people have harmed you or you have harmed another is because of your own soul condition, and you had no control of the emotional errors that entered when you were a child, so do not punish yourself any further.

Learn to befriend and use your anger as a guide on your healing journey. Your anger is your friend, because the more you learn to understand that your anger or irritation is a result of a blockage inside, the more you will be able to understand that every time you feel irritated or angry there is a causal emotion inside you that needs to be released and you are frightened of feeling it. Use your anger, follow its lead, do not project it outwards, but follow it down inside of you until you can access and release your fear of feeling; then go deeper until your causal emotion is revealed.

If you do not feel your anger anymore and you feel emotionally depressed or numb, trace your emotional journey back to how you got to this state of numbness. Follow your depression or lack of emotion back to the place where you were once angry. Between the stage of being numb and being angry is probably a whole set of false beliefs, i.e. "I'll get physically hurt if I am angry" or "I'm not spiritual or a good person" or "God won't love me anymore."

## Emotional Addictions

Another issue that we have to be aware of when we process our emotions is that we do not get addicted to a particular emotion and get emotionally stuck. If you are constantly angry or depressed, then you are addicted to avoiding your true feelings. You are not moving through your emotional process or you are not accessing your causal emotions. If you are crying and crying about the same thing and the emotional charge is not being released inside you to the point where you no longer remember how you felt about the painful event that caused you to feel bad in the first place, then it means that you are either stuck in emotions of self–deception or you are addicted to the emotional pain.

Feeling your emotions does not mean getting stuck in them. Access your causal emotion, then release it and move on. Do not get stuck in the "he said—she said" story either. It is not the retelling of the story or the events that will heal you. It is only the release of the causal emotion that will clear your soul. When you live in your emotions and focus on the story rather than release your causal emotions, you will never lose weight or reach a state of perfected love and become at one with God, free from suffering.

Many times we do not allow ourselves to emotionally process because we are worried about what others may think about us. If people try to stop your process of emotional release, it is only because they are trying to avoid their own painful emotions, so ignore their reaction. Do them a favor by being emotionally honest and process your emotions. This may help to trigger some of theirs. If they try to shut you down when you are crying, simply tell them: "Please do not try to stop me from emotionally processing just because you do not want to feel your own emotions." Let them know that you are doing the right thing by allowing yourself to feel and release your causal emotions. This will encourage them to feel rather than deny theirs.

Letting go and releasing soul errors will break the conditioning that has been imposed on you by your parents, by society, by your culture, and by those unhealthy patterns that have been passed down the generations by your ancestors. Emotions are good; emotions are your guide; emotions are the real you. You should always trust your emotions because whenever you are feeling an emotion, you are accessing information and you are purifying your body, mind, and soul.

## STAYING COMMITTED

There are a series of exercises at the end of this chapter that will show you how to access and feel your causal emotions so you can let go of your grief, your shame, and all of the other toxic emotions that are causing you to put on weight and are damaging your mind, body, and soul. Do not rush your process; be patient; work steadily through the experiences. You have spent years building pain layers and suppressing how you feel, so it will take some time to undo the psychological, physical, and emotional damage. Be patient with yourself if the emotions are slow in coming. They have been buried for a long time, and you have been conditioned to believe that it is a weak or bad thing if you express them. You do not want to replace your deep grief with a blocking emotion of frustration and self-hatred because you cannot do the exercise. Allow your emotions to come up in whatever order they emerge. Your suppressed emotions will soon unmask themselves.

Remember, you can gauge your progression just by your reactions. If you no longer have an emotional reaction to a particular person or event and your Law of Attraction is changing, then you know that you have cleared the emotional charge. If you still remember the painful event, still have an emotional reaction, and still attract painful interactions and events into your life, then this is showing you that the causal emotion is still inside.

There are a number of simple actions you can take to help you process your causal emotions. You may want to write a letter to your parents expressing how you feel about your childhood or journal about your emotions or connect to a childhood home or family haunt. You may also want to take time to look at old ancestral photos or speak to your family about your ancestral history and identify your family patterns. Remember, you do not want just to identify and intellectually understand your childhood, your family blueprint, and your emotional injuries, you want to actually clear your negative emotions and this can happen only if you have an emotional experience.

Before you speak up or send a letter to someone, please process the emotions that you may have to deal with if your family denies what you are saying about your feelings. They may shut you down or cut you out of their lives completely. Be emotionally prepared for the response before you express how you feel to other people. Also, remember that no matter what anyone has done to you in the past, you are still going to be the only one to process the emotional damage inside of you. There is absolutely no use in projecting your feelings onto someone or trying to make that person feel them for you. No one else can feel and release your negative emotions—not even your parents. They may have caused your emotional pain, but they cannot end it.

If you are finding it especially difficult to access your deeper painful emotions, then you can help yourself process by watching a movie dealing with the same emotional issues that you experienced in your childhood or by listening to music with relevant lyrics. All of these simple everyday actions can help trigger your stored emotions.

If you follow the emotional exercises at the end of the chapter and you still cannot feel and release your emotions, then it is not because you cannot access your feelings; it is because you do not want to. You are frightened. Fear covers over the emotional experience of the truth and causes us to bury our head in the sand. Your fear is probably telling you that you are not capable of coping with the overwhelming experience of your powerful causal emotions. Remember that you can cope as long as you emotionally process. The true meaning of F.E.A.R is *false evidence appearing real*. If you face your fear, you will realize that it is an illusion. As the saying goes, "the only thing to fear is fear itself." Befriend your fear just like your anger. Allow yourself to feel your fear—even if you end up shaking on the floor. Let the grip of fear work through and out of you. When you want to finally feel your causal emotions and release your pain, you will. Then you will soon realize that feeling your emotions can be a pleasurable experience and not frightening because with each emotional release comes a sense of purification and relief. Everyone always feels better after he or she has had a good cry.

You do not have to do this process alone. You can ask a friend or a counselor to help you access your emotions by talking out loud about how you feel. Remember that they cannot experience or feel and release your emotions for you, so do not project your feelings onto them and do not get stuck in the retelling of stories. Ask them to hold a space while you talk your feelings through and release them, but only if they so desire. Ultimately, though, it is you and only you who can remove the painful emotions inside.

Another person you can turn to if you want support is God. God can help you if you pray. Say a prayer each night to release your emotional blocks and ask God to reveal your causal emotions through your Law of Attraction. See how different people and events enter your life in the next few days to trigger emotions in you. You can read more about building a relationship with God and developing a powerful prayer practice in Chapter 6.

## PRACTICAL TOOLS

There are also physical actions you can take to remove your body weight, but these should be done only as a support to your emotional release work. There is no use exercising and eating healthy foods if you are still accumulating negative emotions every day. This is why yo–yo dieting or exercise fads do not work because the emotionally rooted cause of the weight problem has not be accessed and released.

While you reprogram your mind, body, and soul and lock in a deep emotional processing routine, it is important to change your diet to healthy, light-filled organic natural foods such as fruits and vegetables. These foods direct from the elements—sun, water, air, and earth—are lighter in energy. They will change the density of your body so it will become lighter and brighter with high frequency energy. They will also provide your body with the right amount of nutrients so the chakra system, body organs, and metabolic system can function optimally. Eat little and often—six times a day instead of three heavy meals. This will boost your metabolism. Also eat a variety of flavors and foods. This not only gives your body a diversity of nutrients but also helps you feel full.

For extra support, love, and care of your body, you should also take a mineral and vitamin supplement to give your system the right amount of nutrients. Our soil has become depleted of nutrients due to overfarming. Many times people overeat because their brain feels starved of vital nutrients so it sends a signal that it is still hungry. Keep your vitamin and mineral intake at the right level and you will not feel the desire to eat so often.

Many people also claim that apple cider vinegar promotes weight loss. It helps to speed up the metabolism, and it burns calories. A number of nutritionists also believe that combining Vitamin B6 and lecithin with apple cider vinegar is highly effective. Many women have found that apple cider vinegar can also help reduce the appearance of cellulite. Fruits and vegetables such as asparagus, avocados, bananas, broccoli, and pears are also excellent foods that prevent the development of cellulite. Therefore try to eat at least six servings of such foods daily. Chives have been known to have diuretic properties; they can reduce obesity and fluid retention. The potassium content of watercress is also great for weight loss, and parsley juice helps the body lose weight because of its effectiveness at dissolving fat and grease which have accumulated in the human body.

If you want to further reduce cellulite, stay away from alcohol, sugar, smoking, and caffeine since these products constrict your blood vessels and may actually worsen the appearance of cellulite. Try to also reduce your salt intake since salt is known to contribute to water retention which promotes cellulite. While you are trying to kick a habit, process which emotions you are trying to suppress with your physical addiction. Process the root cause of your bad mood and physical addiction as you change your lifestyle. See Chapter 5 to learn more about eating a healthy diet, maintaining proper nutritional support, and detoxifying the physical body.

Healthy eating, sleeping, and exercising are all acts of self-love so if you deny yourself any of these in your daily routine, you have issues with unworthiness and self-love that you need to address. Why would you want to damage your body if you love and care about yourself? There is a childhood injury inside of your soul that is causing you to self-abuse. You need to release further unloving causal emotions inside yourself. Self-love should not be about serial dieting or controlling the diet but rather about working through why you desire certain foods that are not healthy for you.

Regular exercise will also help change your body fat into toned muscle. Short bursts of aerobic exercise combined with gentle walking and stretching are particularly beneficial to help you burn calories and lose weight. Yoga is another potent tool. The power of yoga is that it works on all levels whether or not you are conscious of it. Not only does it build muscle, but it is also a very gentle experience to open up the chakra system; yoga allows people to let go emotionally in a safe, nurturing environment. Pilates and weight training are also beneficial. They will help you lose body fat and gain muscles. Muscle is one of the most metabolically active tissues in the body, which means it burns up the most energy. Since your metabolism is elevated by increasing your muscle mass, it is much easier to achieve a lower level of body fat. Free weight training for women can help in maintaining muscle mass so you can maintain a younger-looking body.

Remember to drink plenty of water to replenish your body after each emotional processing and physical workout session. The water will help you stay hydrated and will also help you cut down on calories. When you are hungry, it is often not because you need food but because you are dehydrated. So drink a glass of water every hour on the hour; make sure you properly flush out toxins, replenish what you are emotionally purging, and stay fully hydrated.

Deep tissue massage therapists can also be effective. They can help you release any trauma or grief that is entangled deep in your muscle tissue. Try to find a massage therapist you can trust and relax with. Explain to him or her that you want to release stored emotions from your muscle tissue. At first the massage may feel painful, both physically and emotionally. If the massage hurts, go beyond your pain and allow yourself to scream, cry, and shout. Let your emotions out. In order for the body to discharge fully the pent-up energy from these blocked areas, you must both physically release the tissue of the area and also work through the attached emotional issues. As you clear, so eventually will the pain in your muscles; your soul will ease and you will feel much lighter and looser.

Finally, remember that losing weight does not have to be all hard work and no play. Incorporate things you love to do in your daily workout routine. You can lose weight by going out dancing, attending a rock or pop concert, or by playing hide-and-seek with your children. Look for fun ways that you can exercise and bring the joy back into your life. Just keep moving and share your new body with those that you love.

## CONCLUSION

This is the end of your weight program. If you stay humble and committed to emotional honesty, you will feel and release your emotions and soon see amazing results. When you purge your negative emotions about how others have hurt others, how you have been hurt by others, how you have hurt yourself, and how you have hurt others, your weight will change. Your soul will expand, and your cells will absorb more light. Your body will become a clear, pure light vessel— free of dense negative energy.

Remember that there is no set weight that defines beauty. Release your negative emotions, purify your soul, and your body will naturally return to the perfect weight that God intended for you. From that place of purity you will not only be your perfect individual weight, but you will also be able to feel everything and everyone around you. You will be stronger because you will not only be fully connected to your body, know what you are feeling all the time, and how to process your emotions, you will also be connected to others' emotions. You will become a better friend because you will be more sensitive to other people's feelings.

People will never be able to harm you either because you will always know their intentions and how they feel inside. This means your outer guard and protective padding will further release. You will feel secure and anchored in your own body. As your weight drops off, you will look much lighter; you will move and emotionally express yourself more openly and freely in the world—just as you did when you were a child.

## • *Exercises for Energetic Liposuction* •

The following exercises have been created to help you feel and release your causal emotions. Remember that you do not want to stay stuck in an emotion, but you do want to fully release it. Be patient, take your time, love and nurture yourself through each exercise. These emotions have been stuck in your soul for many years so do not rush through the work or get frustrated.

### Exercise 1: List Emotions Stuck in Your Cellular Body.

* Sit quietly and make a list of all of the unhealthy emotions that you feel are contaminating your soul and are stuck in your cellular body. Work your way through each of the four different types of the emotions stored in you.
  1. How others have hurt others
  2. How others have hurt you (i.e. your parents, peers, society, etc.)
  3. How you have hurt yourself
  4. How you have hurt others

### Exercise 2: Feeling and Releasing Emotions (Sitting)

This exercise helps you experience and purge the emotions on your list.

* To begin the process, sit in a comfortable chair with your legs uncrossed. Keep a towel by you instead of tissues because there may be many tears, and this towel will ensure that you will not run out of something to wipe your eyes and blow your nose! Close your eyes and place your hands on your lower belly.
* Allow yourself to breathe deeply. Feel your belly being pushed in and out. This will ensure you are breathing from your stomach and not shallow breathing from your chest. Open your mouth and allow yourself to hear your breath going in and out—deeper and deeper.
* As you breathe in and out, allow yourself to feel and release any emotions that are coming up to the surface. If you are female, connect with the emotions stored deep in your womb. Speak the truth out loud.

- Remember that as the truth enters, the error and pain will leave. When you no longer feel an emotional reaction or charge, then you will know you are emotionally clear.

**Exercise 3: Feeling and Releasing Emotions (Standing)**

When we move around, we can go even deeper into our emotions to dig out all of the emotional wounds that are stored deep down in our cells. The following exercise will help you purge more of your negative emotions.

- Put on some comfortable clothing—clothes that do not restrict you. Stand up and allow yourself to relax your entire body. Shake your arms and legs, bend over and jiggle back and forth and from side to side. Allow yourself to exhale while you are doing this; push the breath loudly out of your body. Allow yourself to shout, groan, or scream; make any noise you so wish that accompanies your body movements, exhaled breath, and deep dark emotions. Most importantly, don't be embarrassed! You are releasing stored emotions inside of you—fear, grief, anger, shame, etc. If you feel embarrassed, then process the unhealthy emotions of embarrassment and shame. You will begin to lose your weight and your pain if you become childlike and do this exercise. Go on; give yourself permission to express yourself like a child. If you are male—stop being stoic; if you are female—stop being polite. Speak the truth out loud so the error can be released. Experience your suppressed grief. Shout, scream, stamp your feet, and cry until you feel that the frozen emotions stored in your soul and your body have been fully released.

**Exercise 4: Releasing Blocking Emotions**

If you find it hard to connect to your grief and you are still consumed with your anger and rage, then the following exercise will help you to connect with and release your blocked emotion and the emotions of self-denial. You are fearful of feeling the grief so you need to experience the anger to release it and get to your real feelings.

- Find an inanimate object; something that you can punch and hit. Perhaps you have a punch bag in your home or you can simply use a pillow on your bed. Use any of these items: your hands, a baseball bat, or rubber piping to punch the object. Shout your feelings out loud as you are punching. Go on, throw your weight into it—have a good shout.

- Ask why do I have this anger? What is underneath my anger? Speak the truth out loud. Did your mother hurt you or manipulate you? Shout it out loud. Do you hate your father? Has he affected your self-esteem? Did your partner betray you? Say it; get it out of your body. What other unhealthy emotions that are causing you to put on weight have you stored inside of you? How much anger, shame, fear, and hate are there? Beyond this anger, fear, and rage is a deep grief.
- Keep hitting the bag or pillow and stating the truth of your feelings out loud until you are exhausted. At the end of your shouting session, you will probably start crying. That is the place you want to be.
- If you feel yourself still stuck in anger, then keep punching. This may last a few hours or you may have to return to this exercise for a few days, weeks, or months.

**Exercise 5: Invoking Childhood Memories**

- Find a toy or object that you were connected with when you were a child, or look through some pictures of you and your family when you were young, or visit childhood haunts. Feel and release the emotions that come up when you reconnect with the memories of the objects, photo, or place. Once you can look at all of the photos without any emotion coming up, then you know that you have cleared your soul of all of the emotional wounds and errors.

**Exercise 6: Clearing Inherited Ancestral Patterns**

- Discover your ancestral genealogy. Discover the personal stories of your ancestors. Look at ancestral photos. Recognize the similar patterns, behaviors, and addictions that are still occurring today in you and your family. Does your family talk in a healthy way about feelings or are they emotionally repressed? Are you emotionally shut down just like your ancestors or are you emotionally healthy and connected? Are your family's beliefs and behaviors out of harmony with love? Is your family's country of origin an emotionally repressive culture or expressive? Are you replaying your grandmother's or grandfather's past? Are you repeating the same generational mistakes? Do not just understand your ancestral pattern intellectually. End the cycle of generational pain by feeling and releasing your emotional errors.

**Exercise 7: Listening To Music or Watching a Movie**

For those of you still having difficulty accessing deeper painful emotions, listen to an emotionally relevant song or watch a movie dealing with the same childhood issues.

* If you are struggling with painful emotions about your father, watch a movie about a father and son or a father and daughter. If you have problems with an abusive mother watch a film like *Mommie Dearest*. If you have been sexually abused or raped, watch *The Accused*. If you are struggling with your romantic relationship, watch a movie like *The Notebook*. If you are struggling with addiction or an inability to love, watch *Lost in Las Vegas* or *When a Man Loves a Woman*. Select the movie that is just right for your causal emotions. Feel and release your own emotions as they are triggered by the storyline and the characters. Once the emotion is clear, you will be able to watch the film without having an emotional reaction.
* Find a song that reminds you of your situation and allow the emotions to well up and out of your body.

**Exercise 8: Write From Your Inner Child to Your Adult Self**

Sometimes it really helps to put our feelings down on paper. The following exercise is a powerful way to get you in touch with those suppressed feelings from childhood.

* Write a letter to yourself as if you were writing it when you were a child. If you write using your nondominant hand, you will create a childlike feeling.

If you are left-handed, use your right hand or vice versa. This will create a childlike scrawl on the page that will help connect you to your childlike emotions further. Express to the adult you what experiences you have been through and what help you need. Then write a response from the adult you to you as a child; share your feelings and how you are there to love, care, and support him or her.

**Exercise 9: Write a Letter to Those That Hurt You**

- Write a letter to your parents or any other people who have hurt you. Tell them which actions hurt you, how their behaviors in your childhood made you feel, how the experiences have affected your life, and how you would like the relationship to change. Feel and release all of the emotions that come up as you write the letter. You can choose to send the letter or you can burn it and throw it away. You can ask to speak directly with your parents, an ex-spouse, or a friend and tell them how you feel. Before you speak to anyone or send a letter, emotionally process the potential response which may be either positive and helpful or negative and hurtful.

**Exercise 10: Pray to Release Your Causal Emotions**

- Do not feel alone in your emotional processing journey. Talk to a friend, a counselor, or pray to God. Ask for help to release all of your causal emotions.

**Exercise 11: Encourage your children**

- If you are a parent, then encourage your children to talk about their deeper feelings. Do not punish them for their causal emotions. Never spank them—ever. Encourage them to release their negative emotions in a healthy way.
- Do not teach your son to be stoic and strong with his emotions.
- Do not teach your daughter to be ashamed if she feels angry. Do not tell her it is unladylike. Help her move through her anger to her grief.
- Help your children talk about or write their feelings down on paper or to

draw pictures. Hold a safe place for them to fully cleanse their souls.
- Process your own emotions as you experience your children's grief. Your children are your reflection. Everything you see in your children is suppressed inside of you. Your children are teaching you to release your suppressed emotions.
- Observe the adults surrounding your children. Explain the causal emotion theory to them. Ask them to stop projecting their own suppressed emotions onto your children. If they refuse to deal with their own toxic emotions, then keep your children away. The protection of children is a priority.
- If you are pregnant, process your suppressed emotions out of your system. Follow exercises 1, 2, 3, and 4 in this chapter. Get your negative feelings out of your body so your unborn child does not absorb them. Talk to your baby and explain what you are doing and how you are releasing all of your fear, anger, and grief so your child does not have to deal with your suppressed emotions. Eat plenty of alkaline fruits and vegetables to reduce acidity and take extra vitamins, minerals, and omegas to nourish both you and your child. Vitamins, minerals, and omegas are vitally important after giving birth and especially if you are breastfeeding. Many mothers become nutrient deficient and depleted when they are feeding their babies. A lack of vital nutrients causes physical exhaustion and postpartum depression.

## Exercise 12: Eliminate Your Vices

- Cut down your addictive vices such as smoking, drinking alcohol and coffee, or eating sweets and candy.
- When you feel stressed, do not reach for a cigarette; process the emotions, and eat a stick of celery, a handful of nuts, or a carrot instead. Before you reach for a candy bar, grab a piece of fruit instead.
- When you wake up in the morning, do not pour a cup of coffee. Drink herbal or green tea (which is full of antioxidants). Process your bad mood.
- If you go out socially, enjoy your evening without any alcohol. This does not mean you never have to drink again, but it will help you not be reliant on drinking to have a good time. As long as you are processing

your emotions instead of numbing them, then an enjoyable glass of wine is not harmful.

## Exercise 13: Exercise Your Body

- Walk or jog for at least thirty minutes every day to fully oxygenate, stretch, and strengthen the body. Try to make the walk as brisk as possible to burn fat and get your lungs and heart strengthened. Your whole body will feel reenergized.
- Create an exercise regime divided into aerobics, stretching, and weight training/resistance training to build your muscles. Do short bursts of cardio and choose lighter rather than heavier bulkier weights to tone and strengthen your muscles. In order to get the benefits of weight training, train twice a week for thirty minutes each session.
- Do a daily yoga or Pilates practice. Open your chakra system; strengthen and elongate your body.
- Go dancing or to a rock concert.
- Play with your children.

## Exercise 14: Massage Your Body

- Go to a deep tissue massage therapist—one you can trust and relax with. Explain to him or her that you want to release emotions from your muscle tissue.
- Allow yourself to let your stored emotions out as he or she massages you.

## Exercise 15: Nurture Your Body

- Remember to drink plenty of water to rehydrate so your body does not feel hungry. As you emotionally process, you need to replace your emotions with something healing and replenishing like a bottle of water and plenty of rest.
- Eat organic, "light-filled" foods such as fruits and vegetables. See Chapter 5 for more information about proper nutrition and supplemental intake.
- Take a liquid mineral and vitamin supplement to give your body the right

amount of nutrients so that your body metabolizes properly. The nutrients will also keep you from feeling so hungry.

- Apple cider vinegar (ACV) promotes weight loss. Mix two teaspoons of ACV with a glass of water and drink this before every meal or sip it slowly throughout the day. Many women have also found that applying apple cider vinegar topically can help reduce cellulite. Mix three parts of ACV with one part of your favorite massage oil. Gently knead this solution onto affected skin areas twice a day. This massage treatment will help to reduce the appearance of cellulite.
- Cayenne—if you aren't plagued by spicy food, try sprinkling a dash of cayenne on your food. It contains an ingredient called capsaicin that stimulates saliva, stimulates digestion, and accelerates your metabolism at a safer level.
- Seaweed, especially kelp, is a good source of trace minerals. It contains both chromium and iodine. Seaweed is a natural thyroid stimulant as is iodized salt. It is important to regulate your thyroid if you want to maintain a healthy weight. If you suspect your weight issue is due to a thyroid problem or if you currently take any thyroid medication, you should regularly check your thyroid levels with a doctor or alternative practitioner.
- Parsley juice helps the body lose weight with its effectiveness at dissolving fat and grease accumulated in the human body.

### Exercise 16: Crystals for Emotional Release and Weight Loss

- Carry or wear quartz crystal or yellow fluorite. Hold the crystal for thirty minutes every day while setting an intention to lose weight.
- To boost metabolism, carry, wear, or place sodalite or copper in your home.
- For emotional blockages, carry or wear amber, diamond, or peridot to help you release blocked feelings. Place them on your second chakra, (lower abdomen). Muscovite and spirit quartz will also help you be brave and let your feelings out.
- For physical, sexual, or verbal abuse, hold amber or selenite for thirty minutes each day until hidden emotions start to flow. Place them on your second chakra (lower abdomen). Blue chalcedony is also helpful in cases of child abuse.

- Amethyst, melanite, blue quartz, or citrine will help you release anger and resentment.
- Angelite, onyx, smoky quartz, and amethyst will help release grief.
- Ruby triggers feelings of deep pain or anguish, and fuchsite lifts you after you have been hurt.
- If you feel depressed, wear or carry black opal, garnet, sapphire, or tiger's eye and hold zircon so you stop numbing your feelings.

# 4

# Natural Implants

*To be feminine is to become passive, to be feminine is to allow,
to be feminine is to wait, to be feminine is not to be in a
hurry and tense, to be feminine is to be in love.*
**Osho**

Many women, especially in America, are opting for lip and breast aug-mentations to create a voluptuous feminine image. Breast implants have become the social norm. But surgical procedures are dangerous. Im-plants often look unnatural and can easily leak into the bloodstream causing harm to the body. There is a much safer and longer-lasting, natural alternative solution for creating a fuller feminine body shape. It starts by rebalancing and replenishing two different types of energies inside of you.

After you read the above quote by Osho, how did you feel? If you are a woman reading this book, did you agree with the quote and feel proud to be a woman, or did you feel anger rising up in you when you heard the word passive? Did your body become tense with the thought of having to wait? Many of today's women would probably have a strong reaction to Osho's quote. After all, women have been forced throughout history to wait their turn and be passive. Since the sixties and seventies, the women's movement has fought hard to ensure women take action and have an equal place at the table.

So how could Osho, one of the world's leading spiritual voices, make

such a statement about women? The reason is that masculine and feminine are not two separate biological genders but two different energies.

## Masculine and Feminine Principles and Qualities

Both men and women have masculine and feminine energy within
them. The Chinese use the words *yin* and *yang* to describe the energies
that run through the human body. In Hinduism, masculine and feminine energies are known as *shiva* and *shakti*. No matter the different
languages, the cultural interpretations are the same. All humans are
made up of masculine and feminine energy, and each of these energies
has different qualities and principles.

### Some of the Masculine Principles include:

| | | | |
|---|---|---|---|
| Creates that which is new | Extraverted | Combative | Takes action |
| Logical / Thinking | Speaks | Creative | Motivating |

### Some of the Feminine Principles include:

| | | | |
|---|---|---|---|
| Nurtures what already exists | Introverted | Conciliatory | Refrains from action |
| Intuitive/ Feeling | Listens | Receptive | Calming |

When people are operating from their masculine energy and principles, they are creative and like to invent new things; they take action;
they are extraverted and logical. They like to motivate and speak. When
people are operating from their feminine energy and principles, they
are calming and conciliatory; they nurture what already exists, they do
not take action; they listen and feel intuitively. But if the masculine is
not balanced by the feminine, it becomes combative and overreactive.

If the feminine is not balanced by the masculine, it can become too passive and uncreative.

Masculine and feminine energies can be found everywhere in life. Everything in nature is masculine or feminine including our solar and lunar system. There are yin and yang objects, actions, and natural phenomena. Objects with solid, dark, cool, and heavy characteristics are yin (feminine) in nature while objects that are light, thin, hot, and translucent are yang (masculine.) Yin actions are slow and resistant to force, while yang are rapid and move without resistance. In ancient Hebrew tradition, the sun is considered masculine and paternal, the moon feminine and maternal. Similarly, the Chinese believe the sun is made of hot, masculine yang energy that creates and allows things to grow, while in comparison the moon is cool, yin, feminine, maternal energy that soothes and allows for a moment of rest and rejuvenation.

Philosophers have observed that while these two sides are opposites, they are inextricably linked. Yin–yang philosophy encompasses the ideas that opposites balance each other, create one another, flow into one another, and are both required for their mutual existence. If we did not have night and day, the earth could not support life. The same happens with men and women. If either sex is out of balance with its masculine and feminine energy, then problems ensue both for the individual and the whole couple. Our minds are often limited to seeing masculine and feminine as polar opposites, but *shiva* and *shakti* have been married since before the dawn of creation. They are a divine whole that chooses to express itself by taking on the appearance of being masculine and feminine.

God, the Chief Creator of the universe, is also made up of masculine and feminine qualities and energy. We know this because everything in the world is a reflection of God and a result of God's creation. Because each whole soul is created in the image of God and splits into both masculine and feminine soul halves, we know that God is made up of both masculine and feminine qualities and energy. If God was just masculine, then we would not have both men and women as well as male and female animals on the planet or a feminine moon and a hot, yang sun. Nature unequivocally proves both the masculine and feminine aspects of God. Unfortunately this knowledge about God has been lost over the centuries. The feminine energy, qualities, and principles were removed and rejected by Western religious institutions, although many in the East still follow and understand the masculine and feminine principles.

## THE SOUL SPLIT

Unfortunately, most men and women do not understand or even know about these ancient spiritual truths. They continue to focus on the external differences between the sexes and stand divided, battling men against women and women against men. Most often both sexes refuse to consider the opposite sex as a soul and a vessel containing both masculine and feminine energy. They see each other instead as separate, different entities, a competitor, or in extreme cases, the enemy.

The more you clear your soul of emotional blocks, the more your soul expands and can receive more spiritual information about Divine Truth. This will ultimately change your thinking about men and women. You will begin to see a person as an individualized soul with masculine or feminine energy, operating from either masculine or feminine principles and qualities rather than belonging to the opposite sex.

Remember that before your soul incarnated and you individualized into a human form and became self-aware, your soul was, in fact, part of a whole soul made up of both masculine and feminine energy. As I explained in Chapter 1, the soul splits in two at conception. It divides into an individualized masculine soul half and an individualized feminine soul half with each one having its own physical body and spirit body. Each soul half enters either a male or a female body at conception, or if masculine energy is dominant in the whole soul, the two halves will split and enter two male babies. If feminine energy is dominant in the whole soul, then the two soul halves will enter two female forms. This is how heterosexuality and homosexuality occur, and this is also why we have soul mates (soul halves.)

Women are the physical form of predominantly feminine energy, and men are the physical form of predominantly masculine energy although both sexes contain a certain amount of both energies. In some spiritual circles there is a belief that each soul is divided equally into masculine and feminine energy and that we should balance these energies equally inside of ourselves. But I believe that each individualized soul half has its own particular amount of masculine and feminine energy, dependent on how the whole soul splits and how much masculine and feminine energy made up the original whole soul.

Soul halves can incarnate up to twenty to thirty years apart, but it is more usual for soul halves to incarnate only a few years apart. The more adventurous half of the soul usually incarnates first. The second soul half then feels the pull of its other half and incarnates. Part of our healing journey on earth is to reunite the two soul halves and become at one again with God and our soul mate. The reunion of the soul mates helps people attain perfection in love because each soul half triggers the other's emotional injuries so they can heal.

In Chapter 1 you learned that as the two soul halves progress in love, they get drawn back together. They also continue to evolve after they die. When they reach the highest level of love on the Other Side, the two halves release their individual spirit bodies and merge back together as one whole soul. When the two soul halves join together again at the highest level of love, they experience the union of the masculine and feminine and reflect the true nature of God.

To many of you, this information is very new. You may have never thought of yourself as an individualized half a soul. Some may resist and feel that your soul is whole with its own particular journey. I ask you once again to open your mind to Divine Truth. I can assure you that as you continue to do your spiritual practice, clear your emotional blocks and addictions, and evolve to higher and higher levels of consciousness, the soul mate part of your soul will crack open and reveal this truth to you. You will awaken to the fact that even though your soul has individualized here on earth and you have awareness of only yourself at the moment, you are, in fact, part of a whole soul, and half of you is missing. Half of your soul is walking around in another body, either masculine if you are female and heterosexual or female if you are female and homosexual. Likewise, if you are male, your other soul half will be walking around in a woman's body if you are heterosexual and your soul half will have individualized into a man's if you are homosexual.

This soul–mate pairing is perfectly natural and is a perfected system created by God for both heterosexuals and homosexuals. In fact, one of the greatest errors on the planet is how homosexuals are treated. The only real sin is that people do not understand or honor God's perfected system. Homosexuals are perfect sexual beings. Homosexuals are an expression of a masculine dominant split soul or a feminine dominant split soul. Much of the hatred directed at homosexuals is because of a lack of spiritual understanding and a fear of the feminine principles and qualities being expressed between two women or two men. The pervasiveness of homophobia should actually be seen as a pervasiveness of misogyny. Homophobia and the fear of the feminine are perpetuated by people with a deep down fear of feeling and expressing emotions.

Unfortunately, even in today's modern world both sexes are still battling with each other or homosexuals have been shamed into denying their sexuality and so are living a fake heterosexual married life. This means that many soul mates remain separated, confused, and far from God. Most people on the planet are not aware they are an individualized half a soul, part of a whole soul because of their emotional injuries. These injuries block them from feeling Divine Truth. This lack of spiritual knowledge and the intergender wounds that they carry block them from the existence of their other soul half.

## THE SUPPRESSION OF THE FEMININE

The centuries of multigenerational abuse have created a further divide between the sexes. Maya Angelou once said, "The sadness of the women's movement is that they don't allow the necessity of love. See, I don't personally trust any revolution where love is not allowed." Maya Angelou is correct. The women's movement in the sixties and seventies helped liberate women from a life of inferiority and suppression. The movement enabled women to burn their bras and propelled them into the work place. They were able to sit, side by side, with men at the table. But the movement rose up out of anger, not love, and many women became militant and dominating. They castrated the male, punishing him for all that they had suffered.

It is understandable why women became upset after the amount of

# The Soul Split and Incarnation

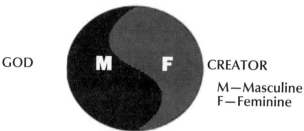

GOD      **M**   **F**      CREATOR

M—Masculine
F—Feminine

God is an entity and infinite Super Being who creates all souls.

A merged soul prior to soul split and incarnation of two soul halves.

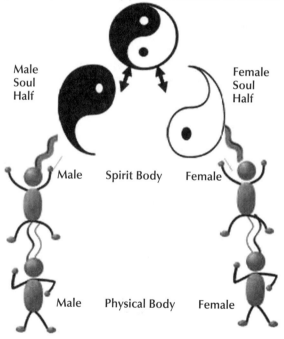

Male
Soul
Half

Female
Soul
Half

Male    Spirit Body    Female

Male    Physical Body    Female

The soul splits into a male half and a female half to incarnate and experience individualization. Soul halves may incarnate up to twenty or thirty years apart, but it is usually only a few. Soul halves are never in the same family. Homosexual souls are created from either a masculine or feminine dominant soul and split into two female or two male bodies at incarnation. The soul-mate relationship helps each soul half become perfected in love, free from suffering, and at one with God.

abuse and suppression they had experienced from men throughout the centuries. After thousands of years of subservience, women loudly and clearly opened their speech centers, but many of them shut down their feeling centers in the process. Instead of processing their grief about the painful things they had endured, they became angry, vengeful, and unloving; they shut down their hearts and lauded their superiority over their male abusers. They began to compete with men and shift away from their feminine energy into their masculine energy. They became aggressive as they let loose their resentment and angrily reacted to how their mothers and their ancestors had been treated. These unloving behaviors, especially towards the opposite sex, were passed down from generation to generation. This shift from passive feminine energy to extreme masculine aggression had a serious affect on women's health and the energy of the world, which was already out of balance because of male dominant behaviors.

For centuries the removal of the feminine has created dire consequences for the planet. The masculine was left alone without the balance of the feminine. This masculine imbalance led to an overreactive, competitive, aggressive, war–like state instead of a cooperative, peaceful, nonreactive condition. We see this imbalance reflected in all areas of our world today. It has caused serious depletion and destruction not only of humans but of Mother Earth.

The earth (Gaia) is feminine in nature, but because she has been dominated by masculine forces, her supply has been seriously diminished—just like the bodies of women. You read in the previous chapters that your internal thoughts and feelings co–create your reality. This means that how mankind feels internally is reflected externally by the earth. Mother Earth is a mirror image of the masculine/feminine battle going on both inside and outside of humans. She reflects the depleted dominated feminine state. She has not been given enough time to rest and replenish. Her resources have been stripped bare, polluted, and destroyed because of masculine competitiveness instead of feminine cooperation.

Unfortunately, today's modern woman reflects the same state as Mother Earth. She is running around doing and being all things to all people. Her output of energy is greater than her input. She is also angry inside, stuck in defensive behaviors. As she competes in a masculine-dominated world, she is consuming her feminine energy. She is emotionally disconnected. She grips and tenses her mouth, her hands, and every part of her body. She refuses to feel and is ready to fight for her place at the table. This causes tension and also creates thin lips and lines around the mouth. Because she is overwhelmed by the complexity of her life, she is so wound up that she is ready to snap. She stays in her masculine energy for much, if not all, of her day. This aggressive energy makes her feel like she is in charge and not subservient to men. But this desire for control actually means she is not strong; she is brittle and fragile. Because she is not feeling her true emotions, she is lost. She is not getting enough rest nor replenishing her feminine energy. This means her body shape is changing, and she is rapidly aging.

What many women have failed to understand is that they are the feminine in physical form. They are born with an abundance of feminine energy, but in their fight to be equal with men, they drain their feminine energy supply. While they raise children and try to be the perfect wife, career woman, and homemaker, their body vessel is becoming tired, sick, depleted, worn down, and prematurely old. Illness, inflammation, hormonal imbalance, and infertility occur because their feminine energy is depleted. Women are burning themselves out. If they are menopausal, their symptoms are made worse because they are no longer a feminine receptor. Those experiencing menopause tend to have too little yin, which has cooling properties. This leads to a relative excess of yang causing inflammation and hot flashes. Menopausal symptoms are becoming even more prevalent in women of a younger age. The goddess is setting her body on fire and literally going up in flames.

If you want to end this self-abusive cycle and avoid painful plastic surgeries, toxic implants, and create naturally a shapely feminine body, curvy breasts, and a full mouth and pair of lips, then you have to move back to living by the feminine principles and replenish your feminine energy. As you refill your body vessel with feminine energy, your hormones will rebalance; your body shape will change and soften, and your persona will also alter.

Hopefully, you now understand that the balance you are looking for is not only about men and women getting equal pay for equal jobs but also about the balance between the masculine and feminine energies internally in humans. There has to be a marriage in every human being of the masculine aspect with the female. Remember that the amount of masculine and feminine energies may vary in each individual soul dependent on how much of these energies were in the original whole soul and how they divided into the two soul halves at conception. But no matter the amount of masculine and feminine energy, each soul half should work towards returning to its original state. Through a synergy of masculine and feminine strengths, we find that the emergence of a whole is far greater than the sum of the two individual energies.

The feminine is the compass; the masculine steers the ship. The feminine is the intuitive, feeling, passive, conciliatory guide who listens and does not take action while the masculine is the logical component of the pairing that creates and takes action. These qualities are not opposites but complements, which is a perfect description of a sacred marriage.

When the two energies are in disharmony inside ourselves or in our partnerships, then trouble abounds; the ship veers off course and crashes upon the rocks. This is why it is so vital for men to embrace their feminine sides and for women to stop depleting their feminine energy. Both sexes, and women especially, have to stop being overly active and aggressive. They have to ensure that with every outward masculine action, they become receptive and refrain from action so they can stop to refill their body vessel. Most importantly, they have to open their feeling centers again, operate from their hearts—not their minds—and compassionately feel instead of think.

The main problem for women stems from the fact that they do not have a clear vision of what it means to be a strong female. There is no model of what is empowered femininity. Even though divine feminine energy is soft, loving, and nurturing, it is not, as many women fear, weak. They hear the word feminine and something recoils deep inside; an image of the 1950s housewife haunts them. They have misunderstood that they need not fear returning to a mute, subservient role because Divine Feminine energy is very powerful and strong—a force to be reckoned with. The feminine is intuitive, all-knowing, all-feeling, and all-seeing. A feminine woman is much more powerful than her angry, defensive sister who is operating from her masculine energy. If the feminine moon is strong enough to affect the ocean tides, then a woman in her feminine energy has enough power to change the world. A true goddess understands this.

Men do not have a role model to show them what it is to embody the Divine Masculine either. The view of the masculine is a distorted one, stuck in ego-driven, aggressive, emotionally disconnected, and power-hungry behaviors. They, too, are in need of discovering the goddess inside them. They need to learn how to feel again and become compassionate, empathetic, and receptive.

In fact, when women first rose up in the feminist movement after centuries of male dominance, many men moved into their feminine energy but became weak and subservient to women in the process. They lost themselves and became confused by what was being asked of them. Even today, many men are still confused and are allowing the feminine to lead, but in the process they have angrily handed over the reins and said, "Okay, you do it all." This is why women are getting so depleted because they get no support. Men also need to embrace and develop their nurturing, cooperative feminine side if they are to become healthy and whole.

There are some men and women already creating new role models of Divine Masculine and Divine Feminine. These people will emerge as new world leaders. They have torn down the invisible barriers and have reunited as one. They have awoken the feminine principles within themselves. When a woman softens and returns to her feminine energy, she starts to feel again, nurture both herself and others, and learns how to listen and receive. She recognizes that she does not have to compete or even participate in the many disharmonious systems in the world that man has created. This is also the case for men who have embraced their feminine energy. They transmit the energy of the Divine Masculine and have gained a strong ability to nurture and feel. They have realized also that there are many systems on the planet that are out of harmony with God's laws and the feminine principles. This feminine frequency will, in time, become prevalent on the planet. When the transformation is complete and every man and woman has healed their

intergender injuries and rebalanced their energies so that they are living from their compassionate, nurturing, cooperative feminine heart
rather than from the intellectual, competitive masculine mind, then
there will finally be peace on the planet.

But how do men and women get to that place of peace and harmony? How do women reconnect to and embody their feminine energy, especially when they have to live in a world still dominated by
men? How do men learn to embrace their feminine energy and how can
women learn to soften so they can naturally create a feminine body shape?

The process begins by doing three actions: *healing your soul mate relationship, clearing your mother and father wounds,* and *balancing your yin and
yang schedule.* If you heal, clear, and balance, your body will become
renewed, rejuvenated, and replenished.

## HEALING YOUR SOUL MATE RELATIONSHIP

## HOW DO SOUL MATES MEET?

If you are struggling to embrace the feminine principles, rebalance
your masculine/feminine energy, and cannot stop looking at the opposite sex as something different from you, hopefully the life-changing
information about soul halves that you read at the beginning of this
chapter has begun to help change your perspective. Hopefully you
understand that you are one soul expressing itself in two different
forms—masculine and feminine qualities and energy.

People long to give themselves completely to someone. We long to
have a deep soul relationship with another human being. This is because there is a spark in us that subconsciously drives us to search for
our soul half or soul mate. At incarnation we are not conscious of the soul
separation—the physical separation of the two soul halves—nor are we
consciously aware of our connection with our soul mate. But the more
we work on emotional processing, the more we will awaken to the fact
that there are two parts of our soul missing—our connection to God
and to our soul mate. We spend our entire life trying to fill those voids
and develop a reunion with God and our soul mate. Until we have
fulfilled these two things, then we will continue to feel discontented.

Soul mates are automatically drawn to each other through their Law of Attraction. Before the world technically evolved, it was harder for soul halves to meet because they sometimes incarnated into separate families that lived far apart so the opportunity for them to meet never arose. For example, perhaps a couple goes on a honeymoon to Singapore and the wife becomes pregnant, but then they return to America. Meanwhile the other soul half of the baby, waiting for its own incarnation, feels the "pull" of its soul mate in Singapore and so it is born in the Far East to Asian parents, never getting the opportunity to meet its other soul half.

Nowadays, most people can travel to any place in the world so the opportunity of you meeting your soul half is much more likely. What you probably do not realize is that you are always connected to your other soul half even if he or she lives thousands of miles away in another country and whether or not you are conscious of his or her existence. In fact, your desires and your decisions will be greatly affected by your soul half and vice versa. There is a personality split between the soul halves, but in God's eyes you are one soul. There will be a synergy in terms of your desires, intentions, and passions unless you have emotional injuries and you are not emotionally open. You are influenced by your soul mate's Law of Desire, and part of finding your soul mate is following your own desires. It is your desires that help you break through emotional blocks; as you clear your injuries, you will find that you feel and desire similar things. This process leads the soul halves back together.

You may even be drawn to go live where your soul mate is. If you were born in Singapore, then you will probably find a desire to visit America or your American soul half will develop a passion for all things Asian and return to Singapore to discover where you both were first conceived. The attraction of the soul mates will draw them together at some stage of their lives.

## WHY DO SOUL MATES REJECT EACH OTHER?

You may already have met your soul half or you may still be searching and confused as to why you have not met him or her yet. There is a specific part of your soul that needs to open to have a soul–mate long-ing. Conscious connection with our soul mate depends on environ-mental factors and is especially influenced by the emotions of the parents. Every single person on this planet has a soul half, so if you are not aware of yours, you need to address the emotional reasons as to why the soul mate part of your soul is not yet open.

So how do you find your soul mate once you connect to your desire and long to find love? If you look for your soul mate instead of process-ing your emotions about the grief you feel because you are separated from your soul half, it will be harder to find him or her. Your loneliness will probably influence you to reach out to the wrong person. Many people attempt to find their soul mates, but instead of attracting them in, they project their feelings and emotional injuries onto other people, believing they are their soul mates. They spend time in a relationship that is based on emotional injuries rather than the love of their soul half. If you emotionally process your grief about being alone, your soul mate will be drawn to you by your Law of Attraction.

Unfortunately, what often happens when soul halves do eventually meet is that they do not recognize each other. This is due to their gen-der-based emotional injuries which affect their ability to know who their soul mate is. The problem is that most people are looking for someone to accommodate their emotional addictions. They think that they can choose their soul mate and that they have more than one, but finding a soul half does not work like this. We have only one soul half ever in our lifetime.

People come armed with a list of ideal personality traits and condi-tions of what they think their partner should look and act like. When their soul mate arrives, he or she is usually not the ideal version; the soul mate is not what the person ordered. This is because most of the traits on the list fulfill emotional injuries and addictions. They want someone tall because they have a childhood injury in their soul about feeling safe and secure. They want someone petite because they have an injury in their soul about feeling manly. They look for an intellectual or someone funny because they want to avoid their emotions or they seek someone with a low sex drive because they have been sexually abused and do not like sex. Whatever their emotional addiction is, they want someone to accommodate it. This is why we will often reject our soul mate.

Perhaps the male soul half wants a wealthy woman with model looks because he has been brought up in a materialistic family where money and physical perfection have been stressed to mean success. He has also been taught to love conditionally by his controlling mother and has set views about the role of women that have been passed down by his grandfather and father. His list of conditions is long, and he is focused on the material rather than the spiritual. Then his soul half turns up, and she is very spiritual; she has not got any money, and she is angry with her father and the opposite sex for dominating the feminine. She has neither the time nor the desire to perfect her hair and makeup. Their picture does not fit—the personality traits do not mix because of their mutual emotional injuries.

Every rejection of our soul mate is based upon emotional injuries. If you do not address your emotional issue, you can come face to face with your soul mate and not know that this is the one. That is because you do not want to address the emotional issues inside of yourself which cause you to reject him or her. The more you can do your soul work and stay open to your emotional injuries, the more likely you will recognize your soul mate. But even then, the reality of who your soul mate actually is can be very hard for some people to accept.

Just think that if everyone has a soul half and there are many damaged people on earth, even murderers have a soul half. In some cases it is going to take courage to reunite with your soul mate. That is why so many people reject the process and try to find someone else. They reject their soul half because they feel it goes against God's Law of Free Will. But remember that God views the two soul halves as one complete unit; the complete soul has free will, not just each half. You are both activating your free will and automatic Law of Attraction when you are drawn together. If you reject your soul half because he or she does not accommodate your emotional injuries and addictions, you will damage your soul condition and stop your progression in love.

## The Soul Mate Union

Even though soul mates may, at first, feel repelled by each other, they will feel an intense connection which they will find hard to pull away from if they are emotionally open. But it is not going to be easy sailing; the soul mate relationship is often idealized. We think we are going to meet and live happily ever after, but you will most likely have intensely negative events happen when you first meet your soul mate. As you pull together emotionally, there are lots of emotional injuries that will be triggered. Soul mates attract in each other to heal soul-based damage. They may, at first, experience extreme highs and lows as they trigger whatever needs healing in the other. For most, the soul mate relationship can be the most trying. They can feel incredible barriers between them that prevent them from having a harmonious relationship.

Your soul half is going to meet your emotional injuries perfectly. He or she will not accommodate your emotional injuries or addictions. But if you keep emotionally processing, then the two of you will keep growing in love and healing together. Unfortunately, most people are not interested in confronting their emotional injuries so they resist and try to find someone else to love. They forget they are meant to be concerned about releasing emotional injuries as they spiritually progress.

You will probably have an injury around the same issue as your soul half but in the opposite way. Take the previous example of the male soul half looking for his rich model wife and the female soul half who does not have money and is focused solely on the spiritual. These soul mates are at the opposite ends of the spectrum. They both have emotional injuries around money, the spiritual and material worlds, and the opposite sex. He is obsessed with money, and she is repelled by it. She gives most of her time and attention to God and wants to be out in the world powerfully competing with men. He loves conditionally and wants a traditional wife who makes him dinner every night. If they both individually focus on what needs healing in their own soul half, they will eventually rebalance each other and heal their intergender, ancestral, and societal wounds. They will meet in the middle and become the perfect whole. They will get closer and closer until they are *One* again—a whole soul perfected in love.

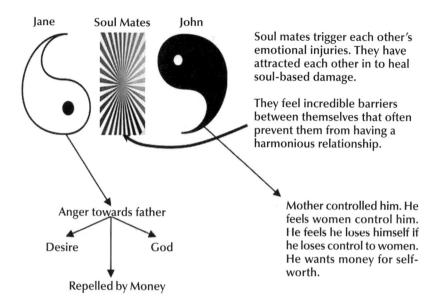

Jane        Soul Mates        John

Soul mates trigger each other's emotional injuries. They have attracted each other in to heal soul-based damage.

They feel incredible barriers between themselves that often prevent them from having a harmonious relationship.

Anger towards father

Desire            God

Repelled by Money

Mother controlled him. He feels women control him. He feels he loses himself if he loses control to women. He wants money for self-worth.

But many soul halves are not conscious enough to understand that the issues they experience in their lives come from their childhood. They do not want to look inside and heal. They blame the other person and usually end up fighting and moving apart. He is angry that she does not make enough money and does not cook him dinner, and she is angry that he is so obsessed with the material world and wants control over the feminine. After months or years of battling, they grow to dislike each other. They turn on each other and start competing, instead of helping each other heal their whole soul. They eventually separate and try to find other partners who will accommodate their emotional injuries and addictions.

They move from partner to partner, striving to be fulfilled. He will probably search for a good-looking model whose interest is also on money and who has issues with a dominant father so she indulges his conditions and masculine anger. She, on the other hand, goes in search of a spiritual man who is passive with the feminine and who also believes that to be spiritual you have to be poor. Their new partners and relationships now feel "wonderful." The new person feels so much easier to be with that it could be mistaken for love. They decide that this is what "happily ever after" looks like. It feels good because they are having their list of emotional injuries and addictions catered to. The mutual addictions make them highly sexually attracted to the new partner.

Meanwhile their soul condition is deteriorating. This scenario can last for weeks, months, or years—that is until circumstances change. The new partner gets pregnant and begins to heal her father issues; she no longer wants to accommodate the angry male, and her looks are not so perfect anymore. Now, suddenly, the male soul half is with someone who is not living up to his expectations; she is also not his soul mate so he feels repelled.

In the meantime, the female soul half has healed her emotional wounds around money; she realizes that to be spiritual you do not have to be poor and barefooted like Jesus or Gandhi. Rather than enjoying her new mate, he does not seem like Mr. Right anymore. As she heals her emotional wounds around the masculine, his subservience to the feminine no longer attracts her. What she sees now are all of her own emotional injuries staring back at her in the bedroom. As she clears her wounds and releases her emotional addictions, the soul mate part of her soul cracks open. She grieves for the loss of her soul half and realizes that the original partner obsessed with looks and material things is her true soul mate, and she loves him like no other.

As you release your emotional wounds and clear your soul, you will soon be able to tell whether the person sharing your life is your soul half or just someone accommodating your emotional addictions. It is only when you clear your emotional injuries that you can find out if your partner is your soul mate. If he or she is not, you will suddenly see your wounded self, and at that moment, the person you are romantically involved with will repel you. You and your soul half will automatically attract each other back when you are both fully healed. If you do deep soul work and activate the soul mate part of your soul, then the Law of Attraction governs that you will not be able to stay apart. Your temporary separation helped heal the perceived separation within your individual selves in order that you become whole again.

You will become the perfect half for your soul mate, and together you will reunite to become your whole soul. She returns to her soft, nurturing Divine Feminine state and balances him to understand that unconditional love is more important than money, and he returns to his Divine Masculine state, at peace with and supportive of the feminine, teaching her that if you have money, you can do a lot of good. As their emotional injuries are released, they realize how similar they are. They become a powerful force in the world through a synergy of their masculine and feminine strengths. Their whole soul is far greater than the sum of their two individual halves.

If you find that you are in this position with your emotional injuries and addictions cleared and are fully aware of who your soul half is, but your soul mate is not aware of you or he or she does know who you are but rejects you because he or she does not want to heal his or her own emotional injuries, do not lose hope of being together. If one of the soul halves does its healing and the other one is still avoiding its emotional injuries and addictions, then the soul will still benefit. Remember that this person is half of your soul and your Law of Attraction. Soul mates are sensitive to each other's feelings. What you do to heal your soul affects the healing of your other soul half. If one is progressing, then the other soul half is being drawn back even if it is not aware of it. As one half of the soul mate develops in love, it is the biggest pull that he or she has over its soul mate. God designed a magnetic attraction between the two souls and that intensifies as one half of the soul pair grows in love.

If you and your soul half are struggling to come together or stay together, then honor your soul mate's free will even if your mate is making choices that harm him or her. Focus on your own response (i.e. your Law of Attraction) instead of focusing on your partner's emotions and actions. If you do not get stuck in blame games and the "he said, she said" story, then you will progress rapidly. Even though from God's perspective you and your soul half are one soul, you just need to focus on the emotional issues of your half of the soul. To clear the blocks, both soul halves must be emotionally truthful. It is your emotional humility (having a passionate desire to feel all of your emotions) that will help with your soul-mate reunion. Keep focused on your own spiritual journey; your soul-mate relationship will lead you to a state of perfected love. You will become at one with God, free from suffering. This will help ease any pain of soul-mate separation. Your evolved soul condition will help you realize that you are never separated from your soul half even if you do not share the same life. You are one soul joined for all eternity.

## CLEARING YOUR MOTHER AND FATHER WOUNDS

In Chapter 3, Energetic Liposuction, you learned how to feel and release your childhood causal emotions. You will find that as you dig deep into your emotional injuries, many of your negative emotions will be towards one particular sex. You have absorbed many of these gender-specific injuries from your mother and your father. You also learned how your mother, in particular, has influenced your soul condition since you were first conceived. Mother emotions are dominant from when we are born. From conception to four years of age, we spend most of our time with our mother. She is our primary caregiver so we are more influenced by her beliefs and her emotions than anyone else. Then between the ages of five and eleven we are sent to school and are taught by predominantly female teachers; nannies are predominantly female, as well. The majority of fathers still work from nine to five, and so our mother or a female figure spends most of the day with us.

If your mother has unloving belief systems about men or is angry and unloving in her actions, then you will have absorbed her emotional injuries in your soul. As you read previously, 80 percent of how you learn to love comes from your mother and 80 percent of your self-esteem comes from how your father treated you. If your mother loved conditionally, then you will love conditionally as an adult, and if you mother did not know how to nurture herself or you, then you will struggle to nurture both yourself and other people. This is why it is vital that mothers heal themselves. They seriously affect their son's and daughter's ability to love and form healthy relationships. Ultimately, it is the wisdom of mothers that will heal the divide between the sexes and bring peace and healing to the planet.

If you are to move back into your feminine energy and heal your injuries around the opposite gender, then you will need to clear the wounds stemming from your mother and father. These suppressed emotions and intergender injuries surface as anger or aggression and throw you out of balance with your masculine and feminine energy. They block you from connecting to God and your soul mate. They affect your soul's ability to return to a place of perfected love, and they affect the shape, the health, and the aging process of your body.

Here is a list of all of the emotions that you need to clear from your soul to help you restore your feminine body and ensure that you are hormonally balanced and in a place of love: *your mother's unhealed emotions towards the feminine, your mother's unhealed emotions towards the masculine, your father's unhealed emotions towards the feminine, and your father's unhealed emotions towards the masculine.*

## THE MOTHER MYTH

As we saw in Chapter 3, emotions around the mother may be difficult to feel. You probably cannot admit your real feelings about your mother or the truth of the situation because, in society, the mother is considered sacred and sacrosanct.

We are allowed to be enraged with our fathers but not with our mothers. We grow up with many myths and revered images of the mother; she is often depicted as a sacred religious icon. "Mother knows best" is the saying—she is pure, good, and unconditionally loving. It is a taboo to speak about mother in less than flattering terms. That is why in this chapter, I am going to focus on the emotions you have absorbed from your mother because they are the most difficult ones to access. Your healing is the key to releasing these suppressed emotional wounds.

This does not mean that you do not have emotional release work to do around your father. You also have to clear your father's unhealed emotions towards the masculine and feminine from your soul. He was also damaged by his mother and father and learned many false beliefs. You have absorbed these multigenerational injuries, too. If your father has been absent at any time of your life or he has been emotionally unavailable or unloving, you will have many self-esteem issues that you need to resolve. If your father is angry with his mother or wife, then you will have been affected by his emotional reactions towards women. As you read in Chapter 3, men, especially, find it hard to connect with their emotions around the father because they are the same sex; they are a reflection of themselves.

Your mother had a group of emotions suppressed in her—some towards her father and some towards her mother. When we look at our partner, we see what our mother feels about her partner and herself when she is with men. We also identify with how she feels about her father. Even a male child identifies with his mother's emotions. He has been influenced by his mother and his mother's rage about multigenerational abuse when men dominated women over the centuries. Multigenerational rage is carried through to each generation of women, leaving an aftermath for the next generation to try to deal with.

For thousands of years, millions of women have been raped or emotionally, mentally, or physically abused. Even if a woman was married, she was often raped. Women have been through generations of fear and abuse. They have also been treated as a lesser person than a man in all areas of life, including most religions. They have been put in a subservient position, unable to teach or lead the flock. In some religions they have been forced to wear restrictive clothing. Their covering is a symbol of invisibility; it is part of the dominance over the woman and the removal of the feminine—including the feminine aspect of God. Many spiritual and religious belief systems have been affected by the society that they sprang from, which tended to be traditional gender-biased, male-oriented communities.

All the abuse has created a huge problem between the genders. There is a wave of rage from women all over the world and a global Law of Attraction that is suppressing women and causing the rage. This rage gets projected onto the child and onto men. Eighty percent of a mother's emotion comes from her rage with men. This projected anger creates serious repercussions for the child as it reaches adulthood. The majority of men on death row come from single-parent families. This is not just because they have low self-esteem due to the absence of a father figure, but because they also have felt and seen their mother's rage with men. This angry behavior then gets played out by the violent son.

## FURTIVE FEMININE BEHAVIOR

When men are angry, they are more overt with their rage; they punch someone, and then it is over. Women tend to suppress their anger, which leads to resentment and underhanded, controlling behavior. Because women have been so terribly dominated and so physically, mentally, and emotionally abused, they have learned an unobvious method of control.

A male controls by force to get what he wants; he is obvious in his dominance. Nowadays, laws have been put in place and he is punished for any physical force he uses. When abuse is physically obvious, we have the emotional tools to deal with it. It is the more subtle, manipulative, abusive emotions and behaviors that are the hardest to deal with. For example, what if your mother tells your father to beat you? Which of your parents is more unloving? Many times, the mother sends a strong message of "You can please me, and I'll protect you because I control your father and he won't hit you if I don't ask him to." Your mother gives the message that she is the dominant person in the relationship and that she controls you, your father, and the whole household. Because of this devious method of control, most people do not tell their mothers the truth.

In today's modern world, there are many men and women suffering from depression caused by a suppressed rage towards the mother because they are not emotionally honest. If you are a woman suppressing anger towards your mother, you are going to end up resenting yourself and you are also going to have difficulties forming healthy relationships with men and other women. If you are a man suppressing your anger towards your mother, then you will either get depressed or your rage will eventually explode in your romantic relationship with your partner.

Most mothers project onto their children what they have not gotten from their lives. Her children will be the people she uses to try to fulfill her emotional addictions. When you stop meeting your mother's addictions, you will experience the fury underneath those emotions. You mother goes from a sweet, caring, loving person to an attacking angry woman. When you go back to agreeing with her, she will be loving.

That is why sons and daughters tend to placate their mothers. They are more prepared to accept unloving behavior from women than men.

The wounded mother wants control. This desire for control then plays out in her relationships. Women who are enraged usually want to find a man whom they can control. If you have a passive man in your life, all you need to do to control him is to be angry with him. Women try to find a passive man who will worship them and make them feel special. But the passive man lying in the bed is like a volcano. He has rage bubbling under the surface that he has suppressed from his controlling mother. If he does not process his real emotions and become emotionally honest, he will eventually become an abuser.

When a woman heals herself and embraces her feminine energy, she does not need to control. She releases her grief instead of her anger. She does not retaliate for the unloving behaviors imposed on women throughout the centuries. She heals her issues with the opposite sex. She welcomes the support and partnership of the masculine. She allows herself to be influenced by him. She allows the masculine to steer the ship as she intuitively guides him. But for this synergistic relationship to work the masculine must have also healed his issues with the feminine, his mother, or the matriarch; otherwise he will not allow himself to surrender to the influence of the feminine. He will still feel like he is being controlled. The male allowing influence from the feminine and the feminine allowing influence from the masculine is the key to a successful partnering.

## How to Heal Intergender Wounds

If you want to heal your intergender wounds and stop damaging your soul condition, it is important that you heal the intergender wounds that have been passed down to you and then to feel and release your grief. If your mother has tried to use control over you, she shows she does not want to feel her own grief about past generational abuse. She also cannot face painful emotions about herself. She carries a whole heap of emotions inside of herself: revenge, punishment, blame, power, control, security, and a need for attention, recognition, and sympathy. These are also emotions that you absorbed and now need to clear from your soul. If you project them onto your partner or perpetu-ate them in your marriage, they will not be resolved. The only person who can release these emotions is *you*.

The problem is that most women often have issues dealing with men's grief. They hate feeling the sadness of the male because they understand that the mother, a member of their own sex, is the cause of it. And rather than wanting to release their own grief, many women have solidarity with their emotions. They speak to their girlfriends about their rage so they can feel stronger. They do not want to feel the grief underneath their angry emotions. Women also deny their fear-based injuries. They have many fears because they have been physically domi-nated. They carry fear of being raped, abused, threatened, or demoted if they speak their truth. They deny these fears and express only anger.

Women have to acknowledge their grief and clear their fears to change their Law of Attraction. But female friends stick together and make pacts to support emotional errors. They create a barrier between their mate and other men. In the feminist movement we see groups of women collectively excluding men. This also happens in the New Age movement where the revering of the Divine Feminine creates women-only groups and an alienation from men, even though men are also made up of feminine energy. The same applies to men. It is their emo-tional injuries that cause them to identify exclusively with their own gender. To remain stuck in gender stereotypes, to defend one's maleness or femaleness, to aim criticism at the other sex for causing problems— these are all denials of the soul's sacred foundation and a denial of the true masculine and feminine nature of God.

Once you have cleared all your intergender injuries, you will never separate the two sexes again. Mature love consists of being able to see yourself in your beloved and your beloved in yourself. I suggest that as part of your emotional release work, instead of putting together a women's group or a boys' night out, you organize a night for both men and women and allow both sexes to speak and emotionally express themselves equally and honestly. As women, we have to remember that the emotional injuries, which have been caused by unloving male behaviors, do not justify our own unloving behaviors as a response.

After reading this chapter, you may begin to have feelings of anger towards your mother as you realize how much she has controlled you and affected your ability to love. Remember not to get stuck in blame and anger and project your emotions onto your mother. This information is not being shared for you to punish either one of your parents. It is to help you clear your grief and hopefully to heal you as a lover and a parent so the cycle of abuse does not continue. If you stay in anger with your parents, then you are avoiding your grief.

Your mother and father were both wounded by their mother and father—just like you. They probably had no idea how much they were harming you. Your grandparents were also wounded by their parents. The damage has been done and only you can heal yourself. These are your multigenerational injuries now so only you can release them. None of these emotions are the truth about the true feminine nature. They have come from intergenerational abuse. Forgive your mother and your father so you do not perpetuate their dysfunctional behaviors. Feel and release your causal emotions.

Commit to ending the cycle of anger and abuse between the sexes. Do not gender stereotype your own children. Try not to dress them in gender–specific clothing or give them gender–specific toys. Encourage your children to play with both boys and girls. Most importantly, do not speak badly about the opposite sex or your partner in front of them. This will affect them later in life. Do not spend time and do activities with your son just because you are the father and do not spend time and do activities with your daughter just because you are the mother. Take turns to spend time with all of your children. These simple actions can make a world of difference in teaching your children how to love and build healthy relationships when they are older.

Your soul mate will be attracted in to you after you have cleared your negative feelings about the opposite sex and released all the false intergender injuries and belief systems. For those already in a soul mate relationship, your connection will deepen and your levels of communication will greatly improve; your feelings will become more loving and harmonious.

So focus on healing your emotional damage regarding love, gender, and sexuality you got from your environment. Follow your own Law of Attraction instead of blaming your partner and reacting to his or her behaviors. This intergender soul work will propel you to a deeper level of purification. As you make a connection to yourself, you will emotionally connect to your soul mate and to other men and women. You will celebrate both your sisters and your brothers. You will return to a healthier, softer balanced state of femininity and refill your body vessel so that it is not so tired, depleted, and brittle. This replenishing of energy will help you feel sexy and receptive. You will move further along your soul's journey towards an ageless state of perfected love. As Victor Hugo said, "To love another person is to see the face of God."

## BALANCING YOUR YIN AND YANG SCHEDULE

There are also practical physical things that you can do to replenish your feminine energy so that your body can soften, refill, and replenish. Our society tends to be very yang; we stay up late, work in stressful environments, and sit for long hours in front of computers. If you want to replenish your feminine energy, you need to rebalance and reprioritize your schedule so it is more nurturing to your soul, supportive of the feminine principles, and the feminine energies in your body.

Below are five steps that you can take to rebalance your life, your hormones, and your feminine energy. Individuals can help promote their own balance through breathing techniques, getting a good night's sleep, food choices, and physical activity. These practices will help your body change. Your lips, breasts, and hips will return to a place of softness, fullness, and strength.

## 1. BREATHING FOR BALANCE

Breathing techniques are a wonderful method for attaining balance. The female body will become softer and fuller when it is breathing in and out deeply instead of taking shallow breaths. Shallow breathing creates a hardened aggressive, "uptight" state.

This tightness makes the body brittle, encourages wrinkles, and depletes the curves of your body vessel. Breathing is mostly a yang activity in which we inhale air into the body to use for energy. By breathing slowly and in a more controlled fashion, we can add yin to the action, thereby balancing out the yang with stillness and relaxation. Breath predominantly in the left nostril is described as cool and is sometimes referred to as feminine. Breath flowing predominantly in the right nostril is described as hot, sometimes referred to as masculine.

Take a deep breath, exhale all the stale air from your lungs, and breathe deeply from your lower belly to release the dense negative energy from your lower second chakra. Contract your abdominal muscles to squeeze out the last remnants. Continue to inhale through the left nostril and exhale through the right nostril while making a buzzing sound, like a bee, with the inhalation. This will replenish your feminine energy.

## 2. Giving and Receiving for Balance

If you want to heal and create natural feminine curves, you need to learn to preserve energy. Every time you do an "outward" action, which means you are in your masculine energy and depleting your feminine reserve, you have to do a feminine inward action to replenish and keep yourself filled with healthy feminine energy.

This means you have to release the causal emotions inside of you that drive you to compete with others, such as insecurity, lack of self-worth, or anger towards the masculine. Then you need to release the emotions that block you from receiving, such as unworthiness, needing control, or repressed anger. This will keep a flow of balanced yin and yang energy running throughout the body. Reprioritize your day so you can have a moment for yourself. Give yourself time to rest, breathe, and nourish yourself after your busy day. A warm bubble bath every evening is a good time to relax and take a moment for you. Put on some soothing music and allow yourself to receive. Release the stresses of the day and fill up with the energy of self-love.

## 3. Sleep for Balance

During sleep our bodies repair themselves and store energy. That is why a good night's sleep is essential for attaining balance. Because the moon is feminine and feminine energy is dominant at night, the more hours of sleep you can have before midnight the more you will replenish. As you breathe while you sleep, you will receive feminine energy. If you have difficulty sleeping, try the above breathing exercise before bed. There is also a point on the forehead just above the center of the eyebrows which can help you relax. Gently rub this point downwards while breathing deeply. Rubbing the ears also helps calm the entire body and promotes relaxation. You may also want to take a walk in the moonlight before bedtime.

## 4. Sex for Balance

Sex is also a good means of clearing suppressed emotions and rebalancing the yin/yang energies. This is why many people will cry after an orgasm. Women especially can clear suppressed emotions from the womb. Sex can be a form of spiritual purification and very healthy for clearing the chakra system if it is done as an act of love rather than an act of self-abuse or a reaction to emotional injuries or addictions. In ancient times sex was seen as sacred–a process of purification and a means to becoming at-one with God. It was considered a spiritual act capable of elevating its participants to a more sublime spiritual plane and level of consciousness. It was never viewed as a shameful sin.

You may have learned false societal or religious belief systems about sex or false belief systems from your mother and father based on their emotional injuries. Unfortunately, many women have been taught to suppress their sexual desire. They have been told that it is unladylike, dirty, and shameful. Then there are the millions that have been sexually abused which has severely damaged their ability to form intimate relationships and love their bodies; millions of others carry sexual shame due to societal and religious mistruths about homosexuality. This shame can also lead to a suppression of sexual desire, an over–obsessive need to perfect the body, or self-abusive, sadomasochistic promiscuous behavior.

Many men also have sexual problems and have been taught to objectify and emotionally disconnect from having sex. That is why so many of them watch porn, seek prostitutes, or develop sexual addictions. They want to avoid their deeper emotions. They view sex purely as a physical activity rather than an emotionally and spiritually intimate sacred moment of deep connection with their partner.

The more you can release your intergender wounds and childhood causal emotions, the healthier your body will feel and your sexual desire will also be healthy. You will have more physical desire for your soul mate. You will no longer desire to make love to anyone other than your soul half. You will realize that the reason you have been sexually attracted to other people was due to your emotional injuries and addictions. Mutual emotional injuries trigger a strong reaction in your second chakra that creates an instant, insatiable desire for another, but this physical reaction actually has nothing to do with love—it is just a reflection of your mutual inner pain. The more you become at one with your soul half, the more you will only have eyes for this partner. You will feel as if you are making love to your partner all of the time—even if you do not engage in the physical act. Your minds, bodies, and souls will become one—a whole soul bathed in love, desire, and divine sexual union.

Learning to love, explore, and enjoy your body is very important to getting in touch with your feminine side. If the lower chakras connected to sexuality are shut down and switched off, then energy will build and create fibroids, ovarian cancer, or uterine problems in women as well as infertility in both women and men. Therefore, it is important to become a receptor—learn to receive and fill yourself up with both the love of God and the love of your partner.

## 5. Healthy Eating and Exercise for Balance

Food choices are fundamental to maintaining balance. If you are low in feminine energy, try to eat steamed organic food. Digestion is a yang activity. Cooking food makes it easier to digest and absorb nutrients.

Both diet and the right supplements provide some of the safest and most effective hormone balancing remedies. The best-researched food for menopausal symptoms is flaxseed. Flaxseeds offer large quantities of a natural hormone-balancing substance known as lignins. Lignins are hormone sensitive; they possess both antiestrogen and estrogenic properties. With regard to menopausal symptoms, they are as effective as traditional HRT in lessening hot flashes and sweating. When you emotionally process, move back into a feminine state, and take flaxseed, you have got one of best natural remedies for taking charge of your menopausal symptoms. Grind up a couple of tablespoons a day and put it in your smoothie, salad, yogurt, or cereal.

Physical activity is also required for maintaining balance. But a proper balance of aerobic exercise and stretching is required. Aerobic exercise is a yang activity. When we exercise, breathing becomes more rapid, heart rate increases, our bodies get hot, and we sweat. Running is great exercise to maintain fitness, but on its own it is often too yang and can lead to injuries. Stretching and soft movement exercises, such as yoga, Tai Chi or Qi Gong, can be combined with short bursts of running to make a more balanced workout.

The natural female body shape can also be enhanced by increasing your muscle mass and reducing your fat mass. Free weight training for women is a way to modify your body shape if you desire to do so. Just like an artist, you can use weights to transform yourself from a woman with a pear-shaped body into a goddess with an hour-glass figure.

For those looking to improve their bust line, there are many bras available to enhance cleavage and shape. The problem is that most women are wearing the wrong bra size. I highly recommend you go for a professional fitting with an expert. Many top department stores have a professional fitter who can ensure you are wearing the right-sized bra to enhance and improve your figure. Enhancing your breast shape through exercise and by wearing the right bra will help you look far more natural than fake; oversized implants do not reflect your natural body shape. Both these simple actions will ultimately keep you safe from the dangers of unnecessary surgical procedures. Remember that the more natural and authentic you are, the more your inner beauty will shine out to the world.

## • *Exercises for Natural Implants* •

**Exercise 1: List Your Masculine and Feminine Qualities**

- Before you can start rebalancing your feminine energy, it is helpful to make a list of all of your personal qualities. Which of the qualities in your personality are masculine and which are feminine? Are you out of balance, aggressive, and competitive? Are you stuck in masculine energy and suppressing your femininity? Do you listen or do you speak? Do you feel or do you think? Do you give or do you receive? Are you too passive or do you need to take action and gain more masculine assertion? Be honest with yourself. Remember that truth and emotional humility leads to healing.

**Exercise 2: Release Masculine Energies and Behaviors**

- Release the causal emotions inside of you that drive you to compete with others (insecurity, lack of self-worth, anger towards the masculine). Then release the emotions that block you from receiving (unworthiness, needing control, repressed anger). This will keep a flow of balanced yin and yang energy running throughout your body.

**Exercise 3: Breathe and Receive**

- Sit quietly with your legs uncrossed. Breathe deeply from your stomach. Work your way through your whole body until each part, each finger, each toe, leg, arm, and your face are completely relaxed. Soften your mouth; let it naturally fall open. Place you index finger on your right nostril and breathe in through your left to replenish your feminine energy. As you exhale through your right nostril, place your finger on your left nostril. Exhale all stale air from your lungs, and breathe deeply from your lower belly to release the dense negative energy from your lower second chakra. Contract your abdominal muscles to squeeze out the last remnants. Continue to inhale through the left nostril and exhale through the right nostril while making a buzzing sound, like that of a bee, with the inhalation. This will replenish your feminine energy.

**Exercise 4: Feeling Feminine Inside**

- Spend the day dressed in your favorite dress or skirt. Choose something very feminine and light in color and texture. Do your hair nicely or wear it loose and natural. Wear minimal makeup with light tones and perfume.
- Walk around your home with no shoes on. Allow yourself to enjoy the feminine feel of your outfit. Fully embrace your femininity. Watch how people, especially your partner, will notice and respond to you! When the goddess is in full glory, there is nothing she cannot achieve or receive.
- If you are male, wear light, loose-fitting clothes. Allow yourself to relax, unclench your fists and your jaw, release your aggression, breathe deeply, and receive. Learn to embody the Divine Masculine.

**Exercise 5: Feeling Feminine Outside**

- Take a stroll in public in your feminine outfit and breathe in deeply. Take the time to absorb the environment around you. Notice as you become present to your surroundings that you have softened. Notice also how many people you attract to you as you walk around in that softened receptive state. Breathe in their love and their support. You are the embodiment of the Divine Feminine; you are not meant to do it all alone.

**Exercise 6: Open Your Heart and Mind to Being Half a Soul**

- Try to open your heart and mind to the fact that you are half of a soul that has individualized. Your other soul half is walking around on the planet either in a male body or a female body.
- If you are homosexual or lesbian, then start to allow yourself to feel that your whole soul was either male dominant or female dominant and split into two male or female halves at your incarnation. Release any emotions of fear, self-hatred, guilt, unworthiness or shame. God made you a perfect sexual being.

## Exercise 7: Connect to Your Other Soul Half

- Make a list of the characteristics of your ideal partner. Do you want someone tall, funny, intellectual, passive, young, black, white, outgoing, Jewish, Catholic, Muslim, Latino, Asian, dark-haired, fair-haired, creative, spiritual, or old? How about someone who drinks and likes to party or someone conservative or wealthy, who owns a nice car or is petite, blond, or sporty? Your ideal-partner list reveals your emotional addictions and prejudices. Your addictions stem from emotional injuries from your childhood. Be honest and emotionally process why the person you want to love must look, sound, and behave like the qualities on your list. Why do you want to be with someone who is exactly like you when you are living from your emotional addictions instead of your pure soul? Do you love conditionally or unconditionally? Are you sexually repressed or physically obsessed? Are you focused on accumulating material wealth because you feel insecure or are you poor and unworthy? Are you biased and looking only for a soul mate of the same race, religion, or social standing? Try to be honest and emotionally release your addictions, judgments, expectations, and conditions so you can recognize and prepare for your actual soul half to enter your life.

## Exercise 8: Releasing Intergender Wounds

This is an exercise to help you clear the grief you feel about how women have been treated over the centuries:

- Make a list of all the things that make you angry about your father and how he treated you. Make a list of your father's belief systems about women. How did he treat women, especially your mother?
- Make a list of how other men have hurt you. Make a list of all the ways you feel that women have been suppressed and abused by men. Speak these hurts out loud until you get to the grief. Repeat the exercises for the emotional release process in Chapter 3 until the grief and anger has cleared.

This is an exercise to help you clear the grief you feel about how women have treated women:

- Make a list of how your mother hurt you. Make a list of how women have hurt, judged, and competed with you and each other. Make a list of how you have hurt other women. Repeat the exercises for the emotional release process in Chapter 3 until the grief, fear, envy, and anger have been cleared.

This is an exercise to help you clear the emotions you feel about how women have treated men:

- Make a list of how you feel women have hurt men over the years. Make a list of your mother's unloving belief systems about men. How did your mother treat your father? Make a list of how you have hurt men over the years. Repeat the exercises for the emotional release process in Chapter 3.

**Exercise 9: Healing Your Relationship**

The following exercises will help you heal your relationship with your soul mate. Be prepared that if your partner is not your soul mate, this work may dramatically change your relationship. These exercises will either draw you closer together or show you that you are not soul mates and just fulfilling each other's emotional addictions.

- If you are in a relationship, start to interact with your mate as part of you, half of your soul, rather than as a separate person.
- Make a list of all the personality traits that you love about your mate and all the traits that you do not love.
- How many similar traits do you have the same and in which ways are you different? Are your differences caused by emotional injuries?
- Focus on clearing your emotional wounds and following your own Law of Attraction rather than focusing on your partner's issues. Commit to clearing only your issues. If your partner shouts or is unloving to you, instead of retaliating, remember that this person is your Law of Attraction. What is in your soul that is attracting that behavior? Is your partner acting like your mother or your father? When did you feel like this as a child? Do you feel unloved, unworthy, or defenseless? The more you can

release causal emotions, the more you will stop reacting to whatever your partner is doing, which will stop the Law of Attraction.

- Make a list of how, when, and why you have hurt your partner. Do not focus on how your partner has hurt you. Remember to ask yourself: "Is this action towards my partner aligned with God's Divine Love and Truth or is this an emotional error?" Ask yourself why did you hurt this person and then set about releasing the causal emotion. Were you fearful that this person might leave you as your father did? Did you feel controlled just as your mother controlled you when you were young? Purge the emotions that come up. As you heal, so you will affect your partner. This person is half of your soul so the love pouring into your soul will help him or her.

- As you clear your half of the soul, see if your list and your partner's list of likes and dislikes become similar. You share the same soul; you will have the same passions, desires, and goals, once you remove the emotional injuries.

- As you remove your emotional addictions and injuries, consider whether you are feeling closer to your partner or moving further apart. Be emotionally honest and humble. This will determine if your partner is your soul mate or just a person accommodating your childhood injuries.

- If your partner refuses to look at his or her emotional injuries and Law of Attraction and if he or she is being unloving, you may need to take some time apart to do your individual healing separately. Even if your partner is your soul mate, you should not allow yourself to be abused. You can return to share the same space again once the abusive behaviors have been healed. No matter what your partner decides to do with his or her process, keep your eyes focused inward on your own emotional errors and Law of Attraction.

- If you are single, then continue to clear your emotional errors, wounds, and addictions so you are ready for love. Grieve for your missing soul half. Keep going with your process until the soul mate part of your soul cracks open, attracts your other half into your life, and reveals who he or she is.

**Exercise 10: Heal the Divide**

- Stop going to women-only groups or boys' nights out and speaking to your girlfriends or your male friends about how you feel about men or your husband or about women or your wife. Start to prioritize and communicate with your soul mate about your inner most feelings.
- Set up a group for both men and women to come together to discuss issues. Be a bridge and heal the divisions between the sexes.

**Exercise 11: Heal the Divide in Your Children**

It is important as a parent that you end the cycle of gender stereotyping and separation. Here are some practical tips for childrearing:

- Do not dress your daughter and son in gender-specific clothing. Dress your children in all the colors of the rainbow so the whole of their chakra system is kept balanced and healthy.
- Stop buying gender-specific toys for your children. Let their individual passions and desires determine your gift giving.
- Try to arrange play dates with both boys and girls.
- Encourage both your son and your daughter to process all of their emotions.
- Avoid projecting your own negative feelings about the opposite sex onto your children. Process and release your own causal emotions.
- Avoid discussing your partner's bad points with your children. Process rather than project your emotions onto your children.
- Make sure both parents spend equal amounts of time with the child/children, wherever possible. Do not over identify with one child over the other just because he or she is the same sex as you.
- Stop comparing your son to his father and stop comparing your daughter to her mother. They are both unique individual souls. Respect their individual mission and life purpose.
- Do not send your children to a same sex school.

**Exercise 12: Practice Giving and Receiving**

- Cut down your schedule. Spend a day doing chores or helping your children; then try to spend some time pampering and nurturing yourself. If you work, make sure you rest at lunch break and do not run errands. Begin to live with the awareness of the facts that when you put out energy, you are stepping into your active masculine energy, and when you rest and receive, you are stepping back into your receptive feminine energy.

- Keep practicing this continuous flow of energy where you give and receive. If you can master doing an action and then learn how to be passive, you will never be depleted of energy.

**Exercise 13: Enhance Your Feminine Body Shape**

- Join a gym or hire a personal trainer to teach you a weight-resistance routine that you can do every day. Remember not to bulk up with heavy weights. Keep the weights light so you can gain small compact muscles. The natural female body shape is enhanced by increasing your muscle mass and reducing your fat mass.
- A very good exercise to strengthen the pectoral muscles and firm the breasts is known as "the lizard." Lie face down and support your hands on the floor to the height of the shoulders. Stretch your arms by lifting the body from the waist up. Repeat ten times.
- Go for a professional bra fitting. Buy a new bra and make sure it fits, enhances, and uplifts!

**Exercise 14: Plump Your Lips**

- The first step to full lips is to get rid of dead cells with an exfoliation treatment. You can gently massage with circular motions on your lips using a toothbrush to remove dead cells. You should use soft motions so that you do not hurt your lips. Natural home exfoliants for lips are easy to make and smooth out your lips. Mix olive oil, sugar, and honey. Take your finger and spread the mixture on your lips.
- For even fuller lips, apply a thick layer of lip balm made of beeswax before bed, and reapply when you wake up in the morning. You will be amazed by their natural fullness.
- Makeup can also naturally create a full pair of lips. Choose a lip liner and

shade of lipstick that complement your skin tone. Choose one more shade that is lighter than the lip liner and lipstick. Line your lips along the outer edge with the lip liner. Apply the next lighter shade of lipstick to your lips, concentrating most of it toward the center. Use the lightest shade to place a small area of highlighter color in the center of your bottom lip and under the Cupid's bow or the center of your top lip. Blot your lips lightly with some tissue. Apply light clear gloss for a dewy look. Put the gloss toward the center of your bottom lip.

- An alternative method is to wear a neutral primer on your lips underneath your lipstick and then apply your lipstick and liner with a touch of lip gloss. This will also give the impression of fuller lips.

**Exercise 15: Hormone Balance and Natural Breast Enlargement**

There is an array of herbal remedies that can effectively restore hormonal balance and help with breast enlargement. You can take these remedies with your omega-3 and–6 fatty acids. Look for these remedies at your local supermarket or health food store or order them online.

- Saw palmetto is one of the most effective herbs for breast enlargement. It is believed that this natural herb is a hormonal regulator and helps in increasing breast size and stimulating sexual desire.
- As an alternative, add fenugreek to your diet.
- Blessed thistle is also an effective remedy for increasing breast size. This herb is a traditional restorative herb that supports the functioning of female reproductive organs.
- Wild yam is a useful herb for various female conditions including breast enlargement.

**Exercise 16: Rest, Rejuvenation, and Sleep**

- Make a commitment to get to bed by 9:00 p.m. or 10:00 p.m. at the very latest. Remember that the more hours you sleep before midnight, the more you will replenish your feminine energy.
- Slip into a warm aromatherapy bath before bed. Massage your neck, breasts, stomach, and thighs.

- For firmer breasts, massage forty grams of Vaseline with twenty drops of essence of lavender. Massage breasts from bottom to top.
- After your bath, slip into some feel-good nightclothes.
- Place a rose quartz, moonstone, or pink agate crystal under your pillow. These crystals will help to soften you, strengthen your feminine energy, and open your heart to love.
- You can also place the crystals on your heart and second chakra (on your lower abdomen) to connect you to the suppressed emotions in your womb. You can also place a large piece of chrysocolla in your home to revitalize relationships.
- For insomnia, hold malachite one hour before you want to go to sleep and put the crystal under your pillow when you go to bed.
- Go to bed early even if you do not plan to sleep immediately. Reading a book will make you sleepy and relax your body.
- Drink some lavender, chamomile, or passionflower tea or use a lavender eye pillow.
- Also, stay away from any electronic gadgets an hour before bedtime. Computers and cell phones affect the production of melatonin, the hormone that regulates the sleep and wake cycle.
- If you really cannot sleep, go for a walk; then return to bed.
- Massage your ears and your temples if you have trouble sleeping.
- Write a "to do" list before you go to sleep so you do not worry about forgetting the following days schedule. Keep a writing pad by your bed for any last minute thoughts or feelings.

# 5

# Youthful Eyes, Hair, and Skin

*We must be willing to get rid of the life we've planned,*
*so as to have the life that is waiting for us. The old skin*
*has to be shed before the new one can come.*
**Joseph Campbell**

You are over halfway through *Spiritual Facelift*, which means you are halfway through purifying your mind, body, and soul. Your rejuvenation and healing process should now be in full swing. You are moving back to a place of perfected love and your authentic self. You have learned about the truth of who you are—a soul that is a container for all your emotions, memories, intentions, thoughts, passions, and desires. You have also learned about God's universal laws. You have read that to stay peaceful you should follow these divine laws and know which false belief systems are causing your wrinkles, mental angst, and disharmony. You have also felt how weighted down your body is with emotional injuries and addictions and that if you want to get to your ideal weight, you need to clear negative feelings that are stuck in your soul. Finally, you have discovered that you are comprised of masculine and feminine energy and have learned how important it is to rebalance your yin and yang, connect to your soul mate, and heal your intergender, multigenerational injuries.

Now you are ready to go deeper to connect even further with your soul so you can live a life of abundance and joy. Mary Eddy Baker once said, "The recipe for beauty is to have less illusion and more soul." It is time for you to discover every aspect of yourself that is still in the dark. As you get more answers and receive more light, you will begin to connect to your soul's purpose. When you discover your purpose in life, your inner joy will rejuvenate every cell in your body.

## HEALTHY EYES

The age–old saying that "the eyes are the windows of the soul" is true; your eyes tell the truth about your soul's journey: where you have come from, who you are, and where you are going. They are a reflection of what is going on inside you—two pools of water that cannot hide any lie. But sometimes those pools become muddied, especially after years of thoughts, feelings, memories, and negative people have trampled through our lives.

If your eyes are not clear, it is a sign that you have mental, physical, spiritual, and emotional toxins in your system. These toxins restrict you from knowing your individuality and the truth of who you really are. They contaminate and block you from living your soul purpose. If you do not live from your soul, then you cannot be all that you are meant to be in the world. Part of finding natural health and beauty is finding the real you. Therefore, to have youthful eyes, hair, and skin, you must be willing to continue your purification process and release more negative things, such as a false identity. This means you have got to look clearly at yourself and tell the truth. You have got to be transparent, look yourself in the eye, and as Joseph Campbell said, "shed the old skin so a new one can come."

You can always tell if people are lying about themselves or how they are really feeling because they will never look you directly in the eye. They will look away, look down, or their eyes dart to the side. These furtive eye movements cause creases and wrinkles. Likewise, if your eyesight is fading, it is because you are avoiding looking at something or someone in your life. If you are nearsighted, you do not want to see the whole picture, or if you are farsighted, you are avoiding what is right in front of you. You want to avoid your pain. As you avoid seeing the truth, your eyes get hazy and out of focus. You start to squint, which causes more wrinkles around the eyes. At the end of the chapter, you will find an array of eye exercises to reduce crow's feet and heavy bags. But if you want to ensure your eyes stay permanently youthful, you have to clear the illusions and open your eyes to truth. You need to ask yourself the question: "What is it that I don't want to see?" Perhaps you want to avoid looking at something unloving inside of yourself or there is someone in your life who is causing you harm, but you are too frightened to let that person go. When you can embrace and stare truth in the face, then your eyes will open wide, and your soul will become crystal clear and focused.

## How to Recognize Truth

In Chapter 3 you learned that the true meaning of humility is to have a passionate desire to feel all of your emotions all of the time. Now we are going to take your humility and emotional honesty one step further. If you want to release your false identity and live from your pure soul, you have to learn to speak the emotional truth at all times, not just to yourself but to other people as well. You have to believe that when you speak and live in truth, you are always being loving to yourself and to other people. It is a basic misunderstanding that you can hurt someone with truth. You never hurt someone with truth. The way you hurt someone is by withholding truth—that is a lie. Remember this: it is when error is leaving people that hurt occurs and not when the truth entering them. If that error was never within you or them, then it would never hurt either of you to hear the truth. If you can expose all the lies, no matter the consequences, you will totally become all of who you are and you will also help other people become all of who they are.

If you follow God's Truth, you will always be honest about your own emotion even if that emotion is shame, fear, guilt, or anger. You will never refuse to speak it in any situation—no matter the consequences— even if you have done something such as cheating on your spouse. You will always state the truth even if others punish you for it. As long as you stay in truth, then you can return to being in harmony with love and work through the causal emotions that made you do the action in the first place. Remember that the truth will set you free as long as you bring your personal truth and your personal beliefs in harmony with God's Truth, which is the absolute truth and not your version of it.

But how do you know if you are speaking the truth and if what others are telling you are truths? Truth has a special quality; it never hurts. It is only emotional errors, lies, and deceit that hurt. Remember that your soul condition is determined by two primary factors—truth and error. Truth and error cannot exist in our soul at the same time on the same subject. You can feel the distinctive energy of truth. You can also feel the distinctive energy of God's Truth. Divine Truth can only enter your soul emotionally; it is felt rather than intellectually under-stood. The absolute truth cannot be realized within the domain of the ordinary mind, only through the heart and soul. But before Divine Truth can be discovered, you have to first face your personal truth. God's Truth is simple. Even a child can understand it. If you are listening to overly complicated, intellectual spiritual theories, then you are listening to truths created by man—not God.

The more you clear your soul of emotional blocks, the more infor-mation you are given about Divine Truth. As a result, your ability to feel and sense things inside of yourself and other people will greatly heighten. With this level of wisdom and sensory ability, you will be able to determine a truth or a lie at any given moment.

To summarize: *Truth* is anything that enters and is retained by the soul that is harmonious with Divine Love. *Error* is anything that enters and is retained by the soul that is disharmonious with Divine Love.

The path to truth is reached by taking four steps:

**Step 1**—Find the truth about God and connect to God emotionally
**Step 2**—Find the truth about me and connect to myself emotionally
**Step 3**—Find the truth about others and connect to others emotionally
**Step 4**—Find the truth about the universe and be overwhelmed emotionally

Unfortunately, many people taking the path to truth never come to true knowledge because at Step 1 they have false beliefs about God. They believe that God is angry and punishing. They do not want to connect emotionally to God for fear of judgment or retribution or they believe that God does not exist at all (Chapter 6 will discuss further our relationship with God.) They then skip Step 2 altogether because it is often too painful; they are criticized and judged by others for processing emotions. But if you can embrace all four steps and remember to *feel, speak,* and *live* in truth, then you will rapidly clear away anything in your soul that is not in harmony with love. This will lead you to your soul purpose and to a life free from suffering.

But be prepared: your journey of emotional truth telling may cause a reaction from others. They are probably used to being able to control or manipulate you or ignore your needs because you hide your real feelings. But no matter what others feel, think, or do, if you refuse to be truthful about your emotions, then you will remain in pain. If you are not truthful with other people about how you really feel, then you will never be yourself in any situation in life. This feels very painful because you dishonor yourself and remain disconnected from your soul.

Remember that if you do not follow the Law of Free Will, then you will always feel others are controlling you, and you will feel that you cannot have your own emotional experience. If you do not speak your truth, it is because you have a desire for approval and you are addicted to being loved.

If you can speak truth at all times, then the negative voices and emotions that have controlled your life will eventually get quieter so you can get to know the real you. You will feel your soul communicating with you and with the souls of other people. From this place of soul-to-soul communication you can start to be yourself with others. You will not want to manipulate anyone or feel addicted to receiving love and approval nor will you allow yourself to be controlled by others. You will simply be yourself and love purely by living from a place of truth at all times.

This emotional truth telling will give others the opportunity to work through their own emotions. Remember that you are also their Law of Attraction so you, too, are their messenger of truth. If you do not tell them the truth about how you really feel, then you deny them the opportunity of processing their deeper emotions. Besides, the more you live from your soul, the more you will feel the pain of any lie you tell. You will feel an instant emotional penalty in your soul. The pain you will feel by telling the emotional lie will be greater than the pain you feel from telling the truth and dealing with others' reactions.

## Truth Never Hurts

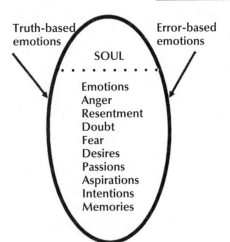

Truth-based emotions

Error-based emotions

SOUL

Emotions
Anger
Resentment
Doubt
Fear
Desires
Passions
Aspirations
Intentions
Memories

A basic misunderstanding is that you can hurt someone with truth. That is never true.

You can never hurt someone with truth.

The way you can hurt someone is by withholding—that is a lie.

It is error leaving the person that hurts, not the truth entering. If that error was never within you, then it would never hurt you to hear the truth.

The main reason people do not speak their emotional truth is that they are terrified of being punished for it. This is because most people were punished at a young age when they told the truth about how they felt inside. They began to feel that they had to lie to protect themselves. As adults we also fear that if people really know who we are deep down inside, then we will be harmed or abandoned. But remember that truth is never harmful. The pain we feel when we speak the emotional truth is only because an emotional error is leaving our soul; it is not because truth is entering.

As you awaken further to who you are and begin to speak truth, you will start to attract or repel different things and different people into and out of your life. You may need to let some people go from your life because you do not feel good around them anymore. These will be the people who do not want you to be emotionally honest. These are people who want to control or manipulate you.

You may find that people want to leave you as well. These people will also be people who do not want to be truthful with their own emotions. They will want to emotionally suppress you and are terrified of people discovering their true feelings. As I discussed in Chapter 3, the more you are truthful and process as well as release your emotions, the more you will be able to sense what is under the surface of any human being. This exposure petrifies some people, and they often go on the attack to defend themselves or to deny the truth. They may leave your life completely.

These people, who live in fear or project onto you, do not serve your higher journey. New people and experiences will soon replace them through your Law of Attraction. They will fill the void. Like you, they will have a desire for emotional honesty and will be more aligned with your new, higher vibrating authentic self. They will be drawn to you like a moth to a light because you will help them feel safe to be emotionally honest. You will be free from judgment, a living example of how to live an emotionally free existence. You will learn more about the importance of letting go of people, places, and possessions in Chapter 6.

Truth talking can take time to develop and become a natural part of you, especially if you have come from an emotionally repressed culture and have been taught that it is impolite to express your inner most feelings. You may have years and years of ingrained beliefs that you need to strip away. At the end of this chapter you will find a series of exercises to help you learn to overcome your fear of emotional truthfulness. Practice on your own first to allow your shame, guilt, and fear to rise up and out of you as you speak your emotional truth out loud. You will eventually find the courage to share your real feelings with others, even if those feelings are disagreeable and do not appease them. The desire to keep your soul purified and to follow Divine Truth will be far greater than telling a lie or offending someone who does not want to be emotionally honest.

Besides, you will not be alone on your journey of emotional honesty for long. Not only is the world entering a new evolutionary era, which is cooperative and intuitive, honoring the feminine and inner feelings, we are also entering the era of transparency. This era has been triggered by the advancement of technology as the Internet and twenty-four hour news cycles expose everyone and everything. Every unethical action is being brought to the surface. No secrets are safe; no lies or unethical behaviors can be hidden inside of us or other people. Even Mother Earth is taking part in this cleansing and evolutionary leap as her natural disasters unearth immoral practices or the harming of her children. Transparency and emotional truth are the future for humanity so we all had better start getting used to being honest!

## THE LAW OF ATTRACTION

Now that you have learned to be emotionally honest, you are further connected to your soul and your authentic self. Now you are ready to discover your soul purpose. Another important part of your natural health and beauty regime is to live to your highest potential and to fulfill your soul purpose. The more you can connect to your soul's desire and break through layers of yourself that have held you down and held you back, the happier you will feel. Your love for your life's passion will raise your energy vibration. Your eyes will radiate a wonderfully free, childlike spirit—the shining light of your true divine essence. The whites of your eyes will become clear and bright, and you will emit a youthful sparkle to the world.

Unfortunately, many people do not live the life of their dreams. In fact, many people do not even realize that deep down inside they crave to wake up every day, jump out of bed, and do something that makes their heart sing. Life's burdens hold them down, and they are too fearful to even try to live their best life. But if you follow Divine Truth and understand God's laws, then you will understand that life does not have to be a burden, an everyday grind, or a struggle. Life does not just happen to you. It is through the Law of Attraction that you can co-create every single moment of your everyday reality.

In Chapter 2, I described some of God's universal laws and shared how many scientists are proving that life does not just happen to us but that we are, in fact, always co-creating with God and the universe. The Law of Attraction is one of the most important divine laws because it affects all the other universal laws of God. The Law of Attraction affects the physical, the metaphysical, the spiritual, and the soul. But what does the Law of Attraction actually mean? It means that the energy of our thoughts and feelings manifests into a physical reality; what you feel deep down inside and what you think about as a result of those feelings creates your reality.

Most people have heard about the Law of Attraction through the popular film *The Secret*. This film taught audiences that if they want a brand new car, they just have to visualize it and it will materialize. Although *The Secret* touched on some truths about this divine law—you can co-create your reality and manifest anything you desire, such as a house, car, job, or relationship—there was also some mistruth in the film which focused only on the power of the mind. The film did not mention how the Law of Attraction is God's messenger of truth, revealing at all times what needs healing in your soul. Nor did it tell you that your Law of Attraction is determined by your soul condition and that your feelings, not your thoughts, are the main basis of the Law of Attraction; everything starts with how you feel.

Every single thing that comes into your life or does not come into your life is the result of your Law of Attraction. The energy of your feelings manifests into a physical reality in the physical material world. When you visualize and desire something, you can manifest it on the physical plane by transforming your idea from etheric energy to concrete physical matter. But if your Law of Attraction is not working properly and you are not manifesting, then it shows you have a problem. What is happening or not happening in your life tells you the truth about your soul condition. It shows what truth has entered and been retained by your soul that is harmonious with love, and it shows you all the disharmonious errors that have entered and have been retained by your soul.

Your soul is a powerful magnet, and as you read throughout the book, your emotions are electromagnetically charged. Your thoughts, emotions, beliefs, and actions attract positive or negative experiences. Every particle in the universe is also electromagnetically charged so it gets pulled or repelled towards or away from you dependent on your emotions and their vibrational frequency. If you send out positive, higher-vibrating feelings from your soul, such as love, gratitude, and abundance, then the vibration of that feeling will attract positive things of the same high vibration into your life. If your soul contains feelings of a lower negative vibration, such as anger or fear, shame or unworthiness, then you will attract negative experiences and block positive things from coming into your life. The more negative the emotion inside of you, the stronger the charge and therefore, the stronger the Law of Attraction.

Your soul condition determines all future experiences, and you can only change your Law of Attraction by changing your soul. People and events will appear in your life again and again as messengers of truth. They will trigger your negative emotions so you can heal them. Their presence in your life shows you there is something inside of you that needs resolution. Once you have cleared the emotional charge, then you will find that your negative encounters stop.

If you can understand the truths of this law, you can take control of everything in your life and progress very rapidly. You will start to notice that every positive or negative event in your life is your own Law of Attraction. When you learn to embrace the truth that your internal soul condition is reflected in your external reality, then you can really start to live the life of your dreams. You are in control of healing your emotions; so if you clear your soul and shift internally, you can change your life into anything that you want.

As I touched on in Chapter 2 when I discussed the Law of Free Will and Law of Attraction, the only people who do not have a Law of Attraction are children because they have no free will. Their parents control all of their actions so children are their parents' Law of Attraction. Remember that the child was conceived in the first place because of the parents' Law of Attraction. The parents attracted in a soul with a particular personality type through their desire. The soul's personality is suited to the healing of the parents' emotions. This Law of Attraction continues through childhood as the child's own emotions and behaviors reflect the suppressed emotions of the parent. The child is the parent's messenger of truth.

This situation will change as the child grows up and gains more free will and becomes an adult. He or she will then start to create his or her own negative or positive Law of Attraction. But when children are young, anything happening in their lives is due to the parents' suppressed emotions or those in their surrounding environment. If your children are angry, shy, throwing tantrums, doing badly at school, or being bullied, they are showing that there is an unresolved emotion inside one or both of their parents that needs healing. That is why the act of spanking is not only abusive, but it is also redundant. As I explained in previous chapters, all you will do by spanking your children is to create a further negative response and to emotionally harm them. The denial of your own emotions through hitting and blaming your children will ultimately cause problems for them later on in life. You will create a causal emotion in them and whole array of capping emotions that will negatively impact their own Law of Attraction. You will also harm yourself because you are blocking the release of your own unresolved emotions.

Perhaps deep down you do not feel confident, so your shy child reflects back your suppressed emotion of unworthiness to trigger your healing and to bring your unresolved, negative childhood emotion to the surface. Perhaps your child is quiet and emotionally disconnected to force you to talk about your inner feelings. If your child is constantly angry, throwing tantrums, or bullying others at school, then he or she is reflecting your suppressed rage, or if your child refuses to take direction from you, then he or she is triggering your own childhood injury of not being listened to by your parents. Whatever is happening in your child's life or you see in your child's behavior is a reflection of an emotion you are denying in yourself.

The more you suppress your emotions, the worse your child will feel because he or she is being forced to feel your unresolved emotional injuries for you. Remember that children automatically absorb all of the emotions in their environment. If you feel and release your suppressed emotional injury, then your child will heal, too, and become more confident, more loving, less angry, and better behaved. The more free will you can also give your children, the healthier (both emotionally and spiritually) they will be. If you are fearful that they may harm themselves if you let them do what they want, then process your own fearful emotions around physical injury or death, and as you feel and release those negatively charged emotions, you will not create a negative Law of Attraction. Emotionally processing this way will keep your child safe.

It can be hard for people, especially parents, to truly embrace the entirety of this concept because it means that they are responsible for every event in their life and every event and emotional response in their child's life. They cannot blame another person or their child or play the victim. Many people do not want to take responsibility for their own emotions or accept that they attract things into their life and their child's life and that they are the only persons who can change their own soul condition.

When you realize that you are the master and co–creator of your life and not a victim, then it is hard to blame other people for your circumstances. Most of the stress we have in our lives is due to feeling like a victim and blaming outside forces for our misfortune. We feel powerless rather than empowered; we become convinced that life is happening to us and that we are not in charge of our own destiny. When we feel like a victim, our mind tells us that we should feel sorry for ourselves and blame other people for our unhappiness. These negative voices grow louder and louder until we have no peace of mind. These stories of victimization and blame block our energy, create tension, and are reflected in a face full of wrinkles and in an aging body. So surrender to this most important of God's Divine Truths because it is actually empowering and exciting. You are the co–creator of your reality, and no one has forced you to be in the position you are in today.

You had a series of desires, feelings, and thoughts and made decisions about where you should live, whom you should date, and what career you should pursue. Before you had decided what you were going to do, these scenarios in your life did not actually exist. You manifested them and acted on every decision that has brought you to where you are today.

You created a *cause* and an *effect*. If you accept the Law of Cause and Effect, you will always try to look at the deep inner cause within you that created the effects you are experiencing. If you do not follow this law and you refuse to take personal responsibility for your own creations, then you will never change your Law of Attraction. You will end up exhausted, and your life will never change. If you want a peaceful, happy life with harmonious relationships, then you must have a desire to clear emotions in your soul. If you are constantly under attack by other people, then instead of complaining about them and playing the victim, you should turn your eyes inwards and look at the root cause of *why* you are co-creating the situation and attracting angry people into your personal space.

You should ask: "What is my messenger of truth telling me that I need to heal inside of my soul?" Once you have that answer and have released the cause, then the attacks will stop. It is not because the other person has changed but because you have released the negative emotional charge inside of you so the other person cannot emotionally hook into you. You will repel that person away from you because he or she will not be able to create a reaction. This person will be attracted to someone else who has an emotional injury or feeling inside of him or her that says: "Over here, I'm unworthy; you can attack me instead!"

Similarly, if you desire material things and greater abundance and you have visualized material things and said out loud, "I want a car," but you still do not have a new car, then you need to realize that your messenger of truth is telling you that your soul does *not* actually want a new car; otherwise you would have attracted it in already. So you have to look at the emotional reason *why* you do not want a new car. Is it because you feel unworthy or guilty? Do you believe that you cannot be a good person if you have money? Or is your desire out of harmony with God's Love, and the only reason you want a car is to feel better about yourself? In that instance, the car will not arrive because the intention of your desire is out of harmony with the laws of Natural Love. Remember that God created universal laws not to punish you but to bring you back into harmony with love. If the car appeared without you clearing your feelings of insecurity, then you would not heal. But if you clear your feelings of insecurity, then the car will probably arrive. Or it could be that you may not want it anymore because you have learned to love yourself enough and have no need to prove yourself through showing off with material possessions. Once you clear causal emotions from your soul, then the object of your desire will arrive in record time. When you release the block, the flow happens automatically as long as it is harmonious with God's laws of Natural and Divine Love.

## Manifesting Your Soul's Desires

Now that you fully understand the Law of Attraction, you can start to manifest your soul's passions and desires. God meant for everyone to live a life of love, co-creation, abundance, and creativity. But unfortunately, mankind changed God's desire to live a life of greed and competition. Humans began to overidentify with the material and physical world, and this created great inequality and disharmony. Passions and desires were cast aside in favor of aggressive dominance and material possession. It left some without—living a life of lack, pain, and struggle—while others acquired too much.

Unless you listen to your soul's deeper desires and allow yourself to follow its passions, then you not only cause damage to your body because your soul is in pain, but you also live a life that is not in alignment with God. Remember that the reason souls incarnate and the reason you were born was so your soul could individualize and gain a consciousness of self. Before your soul incarnated, it was not conscious or self-aware. It incarnated so you could experience your environment and your own free will. Your incarnation also allows your soul to establish personal relationships, develop a natural love for all things in its environment, and develop its personal relationship with God. But your soul has also incarnated to fulfill its passions so if you do not follow your soul's desire, then you will feel unhappy.

Remember, also, your desires lead you to your soul mate. They move you closer to becoming at one with God. You are influenced by your soul mate's Law of Desire, and part of finding your soul mate is following your own desires. It is your desires that help you break through emotional blocks; as you clear your injuries, you will find that you feel and desire similar things to your soul mate. Both of you once shared the same soul so you have the same shared personality and desires. By following your Law of Attraction and your Law of Desire, you not only will find love, but you will also end this cycle of fear, greed, and competition in your own life as you start to create a spiritual existence that fulfills your heart's passions and desires.

But most people do not often dare to allow themselves to feel what they truly desire because of an addiction to being safe. They are fearful or feel too unworthy to step outside of their controlled environment for fear of being judged, or they have been told that they should not have any desires because their mother and father sacrificed their own. They may also feel that making vast amounts of money is more important than following a passion or they feel guilty because their friends are not succeeding. Their guilt, unworthiness, and fear pushes their true ambitions down inside. They numb their denial with food, alcohol, or shopping and do not dare think about fulfilling their dreams.

If you can release these emotions centered around the need to feel safe or in control of your life and stop caring about what other people feel about you, which stems from childhood injuries and addictions, then you can start to activate your Law of Desire and Law of Attraction and manifest a new desire-based existence.

Once you have found the courage to fulfill your heart's desires, you need to know what it is that you want to manifest through the Law of Attraction. The reason many people do not manifest their dreams is that they do not know what it is that they desire; they do not set clear intentions. They have always followed what others have told them to do and never really felt worthy enough to dare dream. They cannot even see or feel what they want to manifest. That is why if you want to reconnect to your passions and desires, you may have to go back to your childhood to connect to your childlike spirit. This is where you can rediscover what it is that you enjoy.

Do you remember what you loved to do when you were young? Did you love to paint, dance, sing, build, design things, or write poetry? That is where you need to begin to connect to your soul purpose. Your soul has a desire and used to fulfill it when you were young, but as you grew up, you became careful; you listened to others' opinions and denied yourself the joy of what you loved. You became so financially focused that you did not dare dream of living your passion.

If you can connect to your original self before the damage set in and suppressed your dreams, you will find your heart's desire. You will know when you have found it because your passions will never feel like hard work. You would happily live, eat, and breathe your life purpose and soul passion twenty-four hours a day.

Once you have found what it is you want to achieve in your life, you then have to set clear intentions, really focus, and feel a passionate desire for what you want. As long as you get clear about what you want and set positive intentions, you can manifest your desires. From this place of clarity and desire, you can activate your Law of Attraction.

There is an array of practical exercises at the end of this chapter to help you strengthen your Law of Attraction and Law of Desire. Make sure you remember that to co-create and manifest, you must focus on your emotions and the level of your desire. Also make sure you welcome your own Law of Attraction as God's messenger of truth about your soul condition and try to remember that your children are also your Law of Attraction. Do not hate, judge, or blame yourself for your own painful Law of Attraction or blame or get angry with others when painful events happen. Learn to enjoy these life-changing divine laws that are designed to help you heal your life and your soul. When you embrace the truth and keep your eyes turned inward, you will rapidly clear your causal emotions, manifest your dreams, and positively change what is coming in and out of your life.

## HEALTHY SKIN

Now you have connected to your passions and desires and learned all of the internal causes of your eye problems, it is time to begin a deeper purification of the physical body. Some of the first signs of aging as you get older are changes to your eyes, hair, and most especially your skin. Just as a caterpillar turning into a beautiful butterfly, shedding our skin, literally and figuratively, is an important part of the process of spiritual transformation. Most women have misunderstood this notion and have spent hours exfoliating, trying to clear and renew their skin. But what they do not understand is that they do not need to burn their faces with a chemical peel or spend a fortune with the dermatologist to have supple, glowing, youthful skin. They can rejuvenate their cells through a deep emotional process of purification.

The skin is the largest organ of the body and requires special attention. If it is reacting, we should listen to it. Like the liver and the kidneys, the skin functions to eliminate toxins from the body, which it does through sweating. Anything that blocks the skin's pores from breathing can cause infections and skin disorders. Once again, we are reminded that we are composed of energy so we should determine what negative, dense energy is contaminating our skin and then set about peeling away the layers and toxins from it.

Detoxifying the liver and kidneys can greatly help to renew the skin. If someone's skin is breaking out, then their organs are struggling to flush toxins from their system; they need to unclog the liver and kidneys. Puffy eyes or dark circles under the eyes can also be caused by the condition of the kidneys. This means you will need to do more emotional release work. The kidneys store the energy of fear, and your skin will break out with rashes when the liver is full of toxins—usually angry ones! That is why it is important that you get in touch with the feelings in your liver and kidney. You need to exfoliate emotionally and release all the anger, grief, and fear that is lurking underneath the skin's surface. Remember that you are what you eat and your feelings are the number one food item on the menu. You need to ask yourself the question: "Who or what is getting under my skin?" Then set about purging those emotions.

If your skin is aging and looking unhealthy, it is also showing you that you need to clear your physical body of harmful toxins. Our skin is a reflection of our inner health, so it makes sense that the more toxins we can eliminate, the better our skin will look. Chemical products and unhealthy foods can alter your eyes, hair, and skin. If you are eating unhealthy junk foods, you need to look at the emotional reason you will not give yourself a healthy diet. When you love yourself completely, you will not want to place anything in your mouth or on your hair and skin that does not nourish or heal you.

Clothes can also harm your skin especially if they have been dry-cleaned; they contain harmful chemicals. Try to use an environmentally friendly dry-cleaner. Hang your clothes by a window to clear fumes off your clothes after you have taken them out of the dry-cleaning bag.

Many of the cleaning products in our homes are also full of harmful toxins that are both harsh on our skin and harmful to our health. Luckily times are changing, and environmentally friendly cleaning products have become all the rage. If you want to maintain your health and skin, you should only use natural cleaning products around the home and natural detergents on your clothes. Nowadays, you can even buy nontoxic natural paints to decorate.

You may also want to wear cotton or organic materials next to your skin. Many people are allergic to materials such as Lycra. There are now many fabulous eco-chic designers who are creating fashionable natural clothing and designer bed linens. All these steps will keep your environment, your skin, and your body naturally healthy.

## THE FOUR ELEMENTS

To purify your body further and ensure that your skin, hair, and eyes will be their vibrant, healthy selves, it is wise to look to nature for support. To function fully the body needs all the four elements—Fire, Water, Air, and Earth.

The sun is our main energy source; water is a proven intelligent, cleansing life force; oxygen breathes life into us, and food from the earth nurtures and nourishes us.

## THE SUN

The sun is our main energy source and not our enemy, but we have been told to hide from it. This is wreaking havoc with people's health because it is a natural source of Vitamin D. Many illnesses, such as osteoporosis, prostate cancer, ovarian, or breast cancer can occur if we do not maintain our levels of Vitamin D. Everyone should have at least fifteen minutes of sunlight a day to feel awake, rejuvenated, and healthy. As you purge your body and move back into a lighter frequency, you will need more sunlight as part of your nourishment; your new body will vibrate at a frequency similar to crystals, and crystals need sunlight to replenish their healing powers, strength, and energy.

The further you live from the equator, the longer exposure you need to the sun in order to generate Vitamin D. Countries such as Canada, the UK, and most U.S. states are far from the equator. People with dark skin pigmentation may need twenty to thirty times as much exposure to sunlight as fair-skinned people to generate the same amount of Vitamin D. If you do not get sun exposure, you will not only create disease but may also suffer from Seasonal Effectiveness Disorder (SAD). A lack of sunlight, especially in the winter months, can cause acute depression.

If you have to go in the sun for extended periods, use a sunscreen with safe and effective ingredients. Most of the sunscreens on the market contain harsh chemicals and toxins so use something natural like aloe vera or zinc oxide to protect and nourish your skin. Many skin experts believe that zinc oxide sunscreen is superior to today's chemical sunscreens at blocking and absorbing the dangerous UVAs and UVBs. In the winter months, try to go for a walk at midday to get your daily intake of sun and top up your vitamin level by taking a Vitamin D supplement.

## WATER

Water is also energy. It is the key to your purification process. Your body is made up of 70 percent water, so as you detoxify and release all of the toxins from your mind, body, and soul, you will need to regularly replenish your body with water. Many people are dehydrated. They have also contaminated their water supply with a lifetime of sugary drinks, alcohol, and coffee. You will need to purify your inner well with pure, clear water if you want to stay young and healthy.

Scientists are proving that water responds to its environment and this includes your thoughts and emotions. Dr. Masaru Emoto, a Japanese researcher and author of the best-selling book *The Hidden Messages in Water*, discovered that crystals formed in frozen water reveal changes when specific concentrated thoughts and feelings are directed toward them. He found that water from clear springs and water that has been exposed to loving words shows brilliant, complex, and colorful snowflake patterns. In contrast, polluted water or water exposed to negativity forms incomplete and irregular patterns with lackluster colors. His research proved that water crystals change, dependent on whether they are in the presence of someone who is in a state of anger or joy. The water crystal structure remains ordered if there is a peaceful environment but becomes chaotic and damaged if it absorbs disharmonious emotions and thoughts in turmoil.

So if the structure of water has been proven to be affected by environment, then think of how you are affecting your body everyday by your thoughts and feelings. Negative emotions change the structure of the water in your body from an ordered structure to an irregular pattern. This irregular pattern causes the water in your cells to change from an alkaline to an acidic state. This change disrupts your PH balance which should be in the alkaline range. The acidity of the water changes your cell structure, which creates disease. Remember, "dis–ease" means your feelings are ill at ease and harmful.

As I spoke about briefly in Chapter 3, cancers cells are caused by a highly acidic body. Cells mutate when the water in our cells changes from alkaline to acid. Cancer cells spread further the more toxic and acidic our environment. Cancer cells cannot survive in an alkaline body. This acidity is being caused by junk food, fizzy drinks, sugar candy, and the chemical products that you ingest or smear all over your body. Yet the acidity is also being caused by your emotions. This is why it so important to your whole internal structure that you remain peaceful and remove toxic causal emotions from your soul so the water in your body does not become overly acidic and harmful. Flood your cells with the emotions of joy and love, and your body will become alkaline and heal naturally.

To keep your body hydrated, you need to drink plenty of water or antioxidant teas throughout the day, especially after you have had an emotional purging session. Drink at least eight glasses of water every day and up to twelve in the winter months. You may want to add a pinch of salt to your last glass as it will help you drink more water. You should also add some liquid minerals to your water. Adding liquid minerals will ensure that the water you are drinking is alkaline. Drinking water from the tap is not safe in most areas. Tap water contains high levels of fluoride and often high levels of estrogen which can affect hormone levels, cause infertility and balding problems for both men and women. Use filtered water only or you can buy a special filter to fit over your tap. You can also buy specialized alkaline machines to transform your water supply into the highest quality of alkaline water. Finally, drink only bottled water when you are travelling abroad to avoid water-borne illnesses and parasites.

During winter there is a tendency not to drink as much water due to the cold so you may want to bring your water to room temperature. You should also leave bowls of water around your house or buy a humidifier to remoisten your skin. Skin usually becomes dehydrated from central heating in the winter or air conditioning in the dry summer months. Do not wash your hands too often either, especially in the winter, and although taking baths and showers is a relaxing activity, your skin may not feel the same way. Hot water can cause your skin to age faster so use warm water, limit your showers to one a day, and limit your soak time in the bath. You should also avoid chlorinated swimming pools; try to find a natural salt water pool instead. I would highly recommend that you avoid hot tubs (Jacuzzis) altogether due to their intense heat and because they are known breeding grounds for bacteria.

## EARTH

Food is made up of energy just as you are—high frequency energy or lower dense energy depending on the ingredients. Food is categorized into two groups: healthy, high frequency "live" foods such as fruits and vegetables that come from the earth or unhealthy, low frequency processed foods, such as canned foods that are created in a factory. Synthetic foods have a dense energy field. They contain "dead" energy that blocks your chakra system. The human body struggles to process the dead sluggish energy through its system, so the food begins to be deposited in certain areas of your body. This causes a buildup of toxins; your body reacts and changes the way it functions. It puts on heavy weight.

You can tell the frequency of food by simply thinking about how close the food is to the sun, the source of life. Leafy vegetables and fruits retain a lot of sunlight so are full of light and high frequency energy, compared to a Twinkie® that is purely synthetic, made in a factory, and denser than our natural state. If you eat foods that are far from natural sunlight, then your body is going to react, and the food, the dense energy, is not only going to be deposited as body fat but is also going to escape through your pores causing rashes.

When you go to the grocery store and walk up and down the different aisles, take time to tune into the energy of the different food sources. You can learn to energetically scan foods and feel their different frequencies just as you practiced in Chapter 1 when you learned how to feel energy. Tune into the different energy fields of the fruit, vegetables, meat, frozen foods, and baked goods. You will be able to tell if a product is unnaturally processed or organically grown. Pick up an apple and tune into its frequency; then pick up a packaged donut. Do you feel any difference in their energy fields? It is important that you eat only those foods that match your frequency and help you feel energetically light and healthy. You should be able to tell if a certain food has the same energy as the frequency of your body and know whether or not you should eat it.

If you choose to eat processed foods, you risk missing out on important ingredients and nutrients, which provide you with optimal benefits. The standard Western diet includes a lot of foods that are low in nutrients and high in acidity such as sugar, breads, packaged foods, and animal protein. As you have just read, the disruption of the body's PH balance not only causes premature aging but a whole lot of health problems. Acidic foods disrupt the body's use of alkaline minerals which, in turn, make people prone to various chronic diseases such as cancer. That is why it is important to cut out sugar and junk food and eat plenty of nutritious alkaline fruits and green vegetables, such as green beans, kale, broccoli, and barley grass to help your body return to an alkaline state.

To restore health, the diet should consist of 80 percent alkaline forming foods and 20 percent acid forming foods. Although it might seem that citrus fruits would have an acidifying effect on the body, the citric acid they contain actually has an alkalinizing effect in the system. A food's acid or alkaline forming tendency in the body has nothing to do with the actual PH of the food itself. For example, lemons are very acidic, but the end products they produce after digestion and assimilation are very alkaline so lemons are alkaline forming in the body. Similarly, meat will test alkaline before digestion, but it leaves acidic residue in the body. Nearly all animal products are acid forming. Figs have many beneficial qualities and help tremendously in alkalizing the body. They can be eaten raw or can be added to any recipe. Dried figs are also alkaline. But since figs are laxative fruits, it is advisable to not have more than a handful in a day. Another fruit that is alkaline is the apple. An apple a day actually does keep the doctor away. Third on the list of fruits that are alkaline are sweet grapes. Grapes are easy to carry and consume. Apart from being high in calcium and potassium, bananas are also alkaline as well as pears, apricots, and peaches which are beneficial for healthy skin and hair. People who suffer from brittle nails will also find that eating fruits that are alkaline helps to strengthen their nails.

If a food source is not produced organically, you could also risk potential health consequences from the artificial ingredients and chemical processes used to make it. If you do not eat organic, then you risk eating unhealthy foods grown on polluted soil. Over the years the soil on our planet has been contaminated by chemicals and has lost vital nutrients because of overfarming. Foods grown in polluted soil vibrate at a low frequency and contain energy much denser than our body's natural pure state.

In our modern world we contaminate our food with many toxins as we put wax on apples to make them shiny or fill foods with addictives so they will keep well past their sell-by date. Our cells are forgetting how to heal and renew themselves because the food source is now unrecognizable due to genetic modification. We have become very far removed from the source of where food is made for our convenience and overconsumption because we have unresolved feelings of self-loathing and unworthiness.

We need to return to traditional ways of eating and to the elements of fire, water, air, and earth. Eating a diet of green vegetables, fruits, sprouts, honey, nuts, and grains will keep your body healthy and youthful. Ancient grains such as amaranth, spelt, quinoa, and kamut are much richer sources of nutrients than conventional wheat, corn, or rice grains. Quinoa is dubbed the super grain because researchers have found that it can contain up to 50 percent more protein than common grains as well as higher levels of fat, calcium, phosphorus, iron, and B-vitamins. Amaranth, a companion to quinoa, was once revered by the Aztecs. It, too, has an impressive nutritional profile. It is high in protein, calcium, iron, and fiber as well as lysine and methionine, amino acids often in short supply in grains. Spelt was mentioned in the Old Testament and is believed to have been first cultivated in Europe some nine thousand years ago. It also tops wheat in protein, amino acids, minerals, and the vitamins B-1 and B-2. It is rich in complex carbohydrates and fiber. In addition to being nutritious, ancient grains also bring dietary relief to people who suffer from allergies to wheat and other common grains. One reason is that many of the ancient grains have survived the centuries virtually untouched by modern plant science. Modern grains, such as wheat are carefully bred—or hybridized—for high crop yields, versatility, and pest resistance. This means that they are now unrecognizable to our cells. Lack of breeding means ancient grains have retained their original properties. They come closer than any other vegetable crop to providing an adequate diet.

You should also eat plenty of fish, soybeans, and raw salads as well as sip natural, healthy drinks such as carrot, alfalfa, or spinach juice along with herbal teas and lots of water. Deadly nightshade vegetables such as potatoes, tomatoes, and bell peppers can cause inflammation, skin irritations, and rashes so limit your intake.

Eating a healthy diet of mostly raw or minimally steamed foods can provide you with antioxidants that will help fight signs of aging. Cooking destroys enzymes, and enzymes are needed for proper digestion. Enzyme production becomes further depleted when we reach our forties, especially in women. If your food is not broken down properly by digestive enzymes, it will cause inflammation, which not only leads to skin rashes but also to illnesses such as arthritis. You may need to take an enzyme supplement to ensure good digestion so your skin is kept clear and your joints pain free.

Most importantly, if you are going to cook your food, avoid using a microwave oven. Microwave oven-cooked food severely damages the molecular structure. Microwaves heat food by causing water molecules to resonate at very high frequencies and eventually turn to steam which heats your food. While this can rapidly heat your food, what most people fail to realize is that it also causes a change in your food's chemical structure. Heating food, in and of itself, can result in some nutrient loss, but using microwaves severely damages its nutritional value. Zapping your pot roast can be a bad idea if you are interested in preparing healthy food. Once again, I remind you to go back to traditional ways of cooking.

As I keep stressing, foods high in omega-3 fatty acids, such as salmon, will produce a hydrating effect from the inside out. In Chapter 2 you learned how these fatty acids help to reduce inflammation, dryness, and the appearance of wrinkles. Skin, hair, and nails all consist of a fibrous protein known as keratin. Keratin production is hormonally controlled, which is why hormonal disorders can show up in nail growth patterns and is also one reason for hair loss and acne at certain hormone-shifting times in our lives. Omega oils and flaxseed meal possess antioxidant qualities and help to balance hormonal levels. This reduces the effects (redness and inflammation) caused by skin disorders and can help an individual heal from a sunburn and stimulate keratin production.

Borage oil is also a little known secret for keeping your skin healthy. It is the richest known source (24%) of the essential fatty acid called gamma-linolenic acid (GLA). The body uses GLA to make the hormone-like substance prostaglandin. Prostaglandin is found to have anti-inflammatory properties. It also protects the skin from damage and regulates water loss. Taking borage oil as a dietary supplement or applying it directly to the skin not only restores moisture and smoothness to dry, damaged skin but can also provide relief to people who suffer from chronic skin disorders such as eczema and atopic dermatitis. Sunflower seeds are also a powerful antioxidant, packed full of Vitamin E that decelerates the aging of skin cells, keeping us looking younger longer. Eating powerful super fruits such as blueberries, pomegranates and acai can also decelerate your aging. So if you want an all-over glow, do not use a toxic spray tan, use flax seed or fish oil daily, apply or ingest borage seed oil, and eat sunflower seeds and super fruits. All these actions will make your skin look and feel better from the inside out. You will naturally acquire a brighter, more glowing complexion.

Even with a healthy diet, I would still recommend taking extra supplements for your hair, eyes, and skin because the soil is depleted of nutrients. For example, as you have already read, the mineral chromium is severely depleted in American soil. Taking a high-grade multivitamin, Vitamin B complex, and some liquid trace minerals containing magnesium, potassium, and chromium will help keep your body's systems functioning optimally.

Herbs and spices can also promote your overall well-being. They are an even more powerful antioxidant than many fruits and vegetables. For example, the organic ingredients found in turmeric can help promote healthy skin. In India and other cultures turmeric has been considered to be a skin food for thousands of years. It cleanses your skin, reduces inflammation, and maintains its elasticity. Parsley is another powerful herb. It contains Vitamin B9, which is a catalyst for the protection of the skin in summer, and it also contains abundant amounts of calcium. In addition, parsley contains folic acid and high levels of Vitamin A and Vitamin C. It plays a key role in strengthening the eyesight and the prevention of night blindness. Parsley also maintains the integrity of the skin and prevents hair loss. It contains a lot of antioxidants; it cleans the body of toxins and prevents the symptoms of premature aging. Basil is also another herb packed full of minerals and antioxidants.

Acne and other skin conditions have been linked to intestinal health, so the use of probiotics could save a lot of time and money spent on high-cost skin treatments. When we do not have proper balance between good bacteria and hostile bacteria in our bodies, we do not absorb fats, carbohydrates, or proteins properly. Nor do we utilize the nutrients from the foods that we eat. When our intestinal flora is out of balance, our system often reacts with acne, skin discoloration, sensitivity, and other negative conditions of the skin.

Antibiotics are a main cause of bacteria overgrowth because they not only kill infections but also the friendly bacteria naturally formed in our intestines. Eating too many sugary or yeast-filled foods such as white bread or sugar-frosted breakfast cereals can also cause a bacteria overgrowth and candida. Therefore, cut down on sugar, cakes, and bread, incorporate a high-grade probiotic into your daily diet, and eat plenty of natural yogurts, especially when you are taking antibiotics. Greek yogurt is especially beneficial at balancing intestinal flora because it is full of friendly bacteria. Not only is Greek yogurt thicker and creamier than other natural yogurts, but it contains more protein and less sugar. Greek yogurt is made by straining the whey off yogurt repeatedly to create its thick texture. Much of the natural sugar is removed during the process. It is also minimally processed and has not been heat-treated. This leaves it full of essential healthy bacteria, including acidophilus. Acidophilus and lactobacillus organisms can improve intestinal health, reduce diarrhea, and help to prevent vaginal yeast infections.

Manuka honey is another natural candida cure and highly effective for boosting your immune system. It is a 100 percent natural, raw, unpasteurized food from New Zealand. Manuka honey is also a powerful healer for your skin due to its antibacterial, antimicrobial, antiviral, antioxidant, antiseptic, anti-inflammatory, and antifungal properties. It should be both ingested and applied to the skin. It can reduce acne scars and heal eczema. In addition, it has the ability to destroy helicobacter pylori bacteria in the stomach which causes ulcers. The benefits of medicinal honey have been known for over four thousand years after the Egyptians started to apply honey on wounds. In today's world, with the growing concern over antibiotic-resistant staph infections and bacteria, scientists are taking another look at honey, especially Manuka and its extraordinary benefits.

## OXYGEN

Oxygen is the most basic element we need in order to survive. We all know that oxygen plays an integral role in making certain that plants and animals stay alive. Oxygen is essential to liberate the energy from food and water for our body's use. It ensures that your natural physiological and biological functions work together in a faultless and healthy manner. Oxygen is vital to your immune system, promotes healing, and greatly enhances your body's ability to metabolize vitamins, minerals, amino acids, proteins, and other essential nutrients. It also cleanses the system, oxidizing and eliminating the buildup of toxins and poisons. Nonetheless, many people do not receive sufficient oxygen to ensure organs remain healthy.

So much of our lives are now spent in air-conditioned rooms in front of the computer that people are not getting a good enough supply of nutrient-rich oxygen. That is why it is so important that we get outside in the fresh air, take a walk for thirty minutes every day, and breathe deeply. Walking by water is especially important. The air around us is filled with electrically charged particles called ions. These ions are either positively or negatively charged. However, the environment we live in today has far more sources of positive ions than in the past. The positive ions create an electrical imbalance in the air and our bodies. Positive ions are generated by heating and cooling systems, televisions, radios, computers, exhausts, cigarette fumes, smog, radiation, and harmful chemicals and toxins. These active forms of oxygen are also called free radicals and are associated with the degenerative aging process and chronic disease. Free radicals steal electrons from healthy cells to neutralize their own charge and thus cause cellular damage.

On the other hand, negative ions have a positive healing effect on our cells. They boost the immune system, elevate our level of alertness, kill bacteria, and increase lung capacity. Water is a great source of negative ions. That is why it is important to walk in the woods, on a beach, near a river, in the mountains, or just breathe in fresh air after a rain storm. You can also buy a water fountain for your home. This will circulate healthy negative ions in your personal space.

## Detoxify Your Body

Cleanses are very popular, and many people like to fast or do an extreme cleanse to purify their bodies. I do not recommend fasting; it can be stressful on the kidneys, adrenals, and other body organs. Drink lots of water instead; cut out sugar, introduce lots of fresh organic fruits and vegetables, and eat plenty of fiber and whole grain foods (such as bran and oat cereals) since they help to remove waste and toxins from the intestinal tract.

Apple cider vinegar is an effective natural bacteria-fighting agent that contains many vital minerals and trace elements such as potassium, calcium, magnesium, phosphorous, chlorine, sodium, sulfur, copper, iron, silicon, and fluorine that are vital for a healthy body. It also helps to maintain a normal PH balance. If your body does not make enough hydrochloric acid, you can suffer from acid reflux because the lack of acid in your stomach is not breaking down your food properly. This is where apple cider vinegar can be helpful. But if your system is too acidic, then baking soda is a powerful acid neutralizer. Half a teaspoon of baking soda in a glass of water will also help neutralize stomach acid. Simple baking soda may also weaken the desire for a cigarette as well as reduce the desire for sugar and sweets. It's used in kidney dialysis to reduce the level of acids in the bloodstream and acts to prevent bacterial growth in food products.

Olive leaf extract serves to remove free radicals from the system and kill viruses. It is recommended for HIV patients to help boost the immune system and to increase the supply of energy in the body. Parsley and cilantro are also natural detoxifying herbs. Parsley is effective for nearly all kidney conditions. It improves kidney activity and can help eliminate wastes from the blood and tissues of the kidneys. It prevents salt from being reabsorbed into the body tissues. Parsley literally forces debris out of the kidneys, liver, and bladder. It cleans the body of toxins because it contains a lot of antioxidants. Parsley juice is effective in dissolving grease and fat accumulated in the body.

On regular consumption, cilantro helps cleanse the body of toxic, heavy metal deposits like mercury, lead, and aluminum. A cilantro pesto also kills salmonella. Chlorella, an edible green algae, appears to bind to heavy metals to both detoxify and remove them. Onion has antimicrobial properties and also helps to remove heavy metals from the body.

Accumulation of heavy metals in the body can hamper brain function, cause memory loss, impaired cognitive function, and Alzheimer's disease. Aluminum is found in about half of today's manufactured cookware. This is why aluminum cookware should be avoided. There are medical concerns that toxic levels of aluminum could be absorbed into the body when cooking with the metal. The intake of too much aluminum has not only been linked to Alzheimer's disease, but it might also impair the kidneys, which excrete the metal. Toxic levels of aluminum may cause anemia, decreased liver function, poor coordination, calcium deficiency, and memory loss among other health issues. Aluminum is almost everywhere in our environment. It can found in our air and water and in many medicines. The average person takes in anywhere from 3 to 50 mg of aluminum each day, but people can expect to ingest 3 to 6 mg each time they cook with aluminum pots and pans. Despite these health hazards, aluminum cookware remains popular because it is lightweight, low-priced, and a powerful heat conductor. But aluminum is also highly reactive. Cooking acidic foods such as tomatoes can cause leaching. The food actually absorbs the aluminum from the pot or pan, which means that you will be swallowing aluminum particles from the cookware. Therefore, avoid cooking acidic foods in aluminum cookware and do not store foods in aluminum containers. To ensure your body is protected from high levels of aluminum, use cast-iron, glass, or stainless steel pots and pans as an alternative. Do not use aluminum foil either. Instead, try using parchment paper—also called baking paper. It is moisture resistant, grease resistant, and makes cleaning up easy.

Aluminum is also present in some personal care products. It is important that you use a natural deodorant that does not contain aluminum. It has been suggested that deodorants maybe linked to breast cancer.

We are also consuming mercury more than ever because of the high levels in sea water and because of a trend in eating sushi. We are also carrying a lot of mercury around in our mouths. Mercury fillings can seep into the body and create serious health issues. Symptoms associated with mercury contamination include Alzheimer's, kidney dysfunction, multiple sclerosis, and thyroid problems. The list is growing as more studies are done. The brain, central nervous system, and fatty tissues are the main areas in the body where mercury is stored. Our body is capable of excreting mercury, however only in small amounts so mercury fillings cause the mercury levels in the body to rise in excess of our ability to excrete it. Therefore, our body stores it because there is nowhere else for it to go.

The term "Mad as a Hatter" did not originate from Lewis Carroll. In 1837 it was believed that hatters really did go mad. The chemicals used in hat-making included mercurous nitrate, used in curing felt. Prolonged exposure to the mercury vapors caused mercury poisoning. The older hat makers developed severe and uncontrollable muscular tremors and twitching limbs, called "hatter's shakes." Other symptoms included distorted vision and confused speech while more advanced cases developed hallucinations and other psychotic symptoms.

So why have we been putting this toxic substance in our mouths and the mouths of our children? The toxicity of mercury has never been in question. The real question is what are the possible consequences for our children at low doses? Autism advocates are especially concerned about the amounts of mercury being used in vaccinations. They recommend that if parents are going to have their child vaccinated, then they should keep the vaccinations to an absolute minimum and do not do too many at one time so the child's sensitive system does not get overloaded with heavy metals and toxins. If you have questions about your child's immunity, research further on this important subject and consult your child's physician.

An important part of your detoxification process should be to find a holistic dentist, who specializes in removing mercury fillings. Many dentists still refuse to acknowledge the dangers of mercury and do not take extra precaution when removing fillings. If your dentist does not insist you wear an oxygen mask and have a constant drain in your mouth to remove the toxic metal he is drilling so it does not enter your digestive and nervous system, then please find another dentist who is an expert on working with this life-threatening material.

Many name-brand toothpastes and mouthwashes also contain potentially harmful ingredients that can penetrate through the tissue of your mouth, enter your blood stream, and build up in your liver, kidneys, heart, lungs, and tissues. Just read the label on any major brand toothpaste or mouthwash and you will see they are loaded with dangerous toxins and chemicals such as sodium fluoride, triclosan, FD&C Blue Dye #1 and #2, sodium lauryl sulfate, and hydrated silica. All of these common ingredients have been found to be harmful to humans. Sodium fluoride is one of the main ingredients in rat poison and FD&C Blue Dye #1 and #2 are just like ingesting crude oil as they are synthesized from petroleum. Perhaps the most dangerous ingredient in toothpaste is sodium lauryl sulfate (SLS). SLS is added to toothpastes and other personal-care products such as shampoos in order to generate foam and to give the impression that the product is working. But sodium lauryl sulfate is very strong, and it is also used in products such as garage-floor cleaners, engine degreasers, and car-wash soaps. Another toxic chemical in toothpaste and mouthwash is triclosan. This chemical is also found in antibacterial soaps, shaving creams, deodorants, first-aid creams, kitchenware, clothes, and toys. Triclosan kills bacteria; that is why it is used in so many hand soaps, but research has shown that prominent bacteria such as e. coli, salmonella, and other intestinal bacteria become resistant to triclosan pretty quickly. But there are other concerns that it is an endocrine disruptor and may interfere with normal functioning of your thyroid hormone and estrogen. It may also trigger allergies.

Many toothpaste brands also use hydrated silica as a whitener, but this abrasive is made from a crystallized compound found in flint and sand which harms the enamel. While silica can remove tartar and make teeth whiter, it also alters the acidic balance of the mouth, gums, and tongue which can cause dental decay. That is why I highly recommend, you buy an all-natural alternative toothpaste. Baking soda is especially good for whitening teeth and reducing acidity in the mouth. A sprig of parsley is also beneficial for keeping breath fresh. There is continuous controversy regarding the use of fluoride or non-fluoride toothpaste and whether fluoride should or should not be in our water supply so I leave it to you to decide. Most dentists state that fluoride is necessary for the health of teeth but according to the handbook *Clinical Toxicology of Commercial Products* fluoride is more poisonous than lead and just slightly less poisonous than arsenic.[1] It is a cumulative poison that builds up in bone over the years. That is why many people prefer to avoid ingesting fluoride altogether.

Some people also choose to remove shellfish from their diet. Shellfish are known "bottom feeders." Crustaceans are scavengers; they feed on scraps and dead creatures at the bottom of the ocean. This means shellfish can contain an abundance of bacteria and even parasites. If you are going to eat shellfish, ensure that you also eat garlic. Garlic is a known killer of parasites.

[1]Marion N. Gleason, Robert E. Gosselin, and Harold C. Hodge, *Clinical Toxicology of Commercial Products: Acute Poisoning (Home & Farm)* ( Baltimore: The Williams & Wilkins Co., 1957), 143-44.

But as I have stressed through this book, the most important thing you can do to detoxify your body is to emotionally process. As long as you are doing your emotional processing work as part of your health regime, your body will natural cleanse itself from the inside out.

## HEALTHY HAIR

Eating a healthy diet is not only the most important thing you can do for your eyes and skin but also for your hair. The main cause of hair problems is unhealthy junk food. If you do not ingest the correct amount of nutrients, then your hair will start to break, grow thin, and turn grey. If you want to maintain a full head of glossy, strong hair throughout your older years, you need a daily intake of vitamins and minerals through eating a healthy diet and taking supplements. Iron is an essential mineral for hair health. Good sources of iron in your diet include: liver, beef, fish, leafy greens, fortified cereal, beans, and pumpkin seeds. Vitamin C foods help in the absorption of iron. Try to combine the iron source with a Vitamin C source at the same time. Good sources of Vitamin C include: citrus fruit, green leafy vegetables, and tomatoes.

A deficiency in protein can also lead to hair loss; adequate protein can help to provide the amino acids that strengthen hair. Good sources of protein include: seafood, white-meat poultry, milk, cheese, yogurt, eggs, beans, and soy. Vegans can get good nonanimal protein from tofu, whole-wheat bread, peanut butter, brown rice, lentils, quinoa, nuts, beans, and broccoli. Omega fats keep hair healthy and have a role in preventing hair from becoming dry and brittle. Biotin, a B vitamin, is also important for healthy hair. Good sources of biotin include: brewer's yeast, bulgur wheat, lentils, sunflower seeds, soybeans, and walnuts. Zinc is important for hair nourishment, too. Drinking lots of water, along with fresh juices such as carrot or spinach, is also good for health and hair.

Other major causes of hair breakage and hair loss are hormone imbalance, pollution, genetics, emotional stress, and depression. Many women lose their hair due to thyroid problems. Low thyroid levels also cause skin rashes so it is important to maintain your iodine levels with natural sources such as sea foods, iodized salt, or sea vegetables such as kelp. Some people also choose to take an iodine supplement. In the 1960s bread used to contain iodine, but due to health concerns a decision was made twenty years ago to remove iodine from bread and replace it with bromine. Since then levels of iodine have fallen by 50 percent even though iodine is an essential element in the production of thyroid hormones by the thyroid gland. The breasts are the second main glandular storage site for iodine. That is why I believe it is vital we maintain our levels of iodine to prevent thyroid disease and breast cancer. Some of the thyroid medications on the market can cause extra hair loss so taking a natural form of iodine can be just as effective in normalizing thyroid levels without causing harmful side effects. But as I mentioned in Chapter 3, when you introduce foods such as kelp to your diet or an iodine supplement, keep a check on your thyroid levels and have regular checkups with your doctor.

Hair loss is also prevalent because of stress. As you simplify your life and release harmful people and things, you will de-stress. This will greatly affect the health of your hair. The body is literally "pulling" its hair out, splitting itself in two, and crying for your attention. If people can slow down, their hair will stop falling. If you take a high grade Vitamin B, then your stress will decrease. Some claim that a PABA supplement (para-aminobenzoic acid) also reduces stress and promotes both healthy skin and hair growth. It can also help to restore hair loss and restore hair color. PABA is found in liver, brewer's yeast, wheat germ, whole grains, and eggs.

Other causes of thinning or badly conditioned lackluster hair are excessive consumption of caffeine, alcohol, and the side effects of prescription drugs. Other culprits are all the styling products that we regularly use. They are full of chemicals that strip our hair of natural oils and take away its natural shine. Most commercial shampoos contain those harmful lather-rich sulfates that are also present in toothpaste. They do more damage than good. It is also important to avoid using chemical-based bleach, hair color, or hair gels as they contain ammonia. These chemical products build up in your hair which dulls the natural gloss and tone of your hair. Excessive heat such as using hair curlers, flat irons, and hair dryers also greatly damage your hair. It becomes dry, lifeless, and hard.

To revitalize hair and keep it looking young and healthy, you need a regular, natural hair-care routine. Regularly cleaning your hair with natural, sulfate-free shampoos containing vitamins, minerals, and natural oils is important. Also using a shampoo containing biotin helps nourish hair and reduces hair loss. Keratin shampoo helps to repair and strengthen hair, enhance its elasticity, and reduce breakage while cleansing the hair and scalp. Regular trimming prevents split ends and keeps it strong while head massages activate sebaceous glands. Their secretions make your hair strong and shiny as they promote blood circulation and prevent hair loss. You can massage your hair and scalp simply with your hand, or you can use coconut or warm olive oil.

There are many useful home remedies for hair care that nourish hair without side effects; these can help your hair bounce and shine with good health. You can get rid of the buildup of chemicals by applying a mix of apple cider vinegar and distilled water or use lime juice as a cleanser. Another great tip is to use baking soda once a week mixed with your shampoo to strip off a build-up of products.

If you can reduce your stress, process your emotional pain, eat a healthy diet, manage your hormonal levels, and avoid chemical products, then your hair will reflect your natural health and inner beauty; you will prevent breakage and hair loss while having a lifetime of glossy, healthy hair.

## CONCLUSION

Now that you are fully connected to your soul and you have discovered your soul purpose, you have found beauty because you have found the real you.

As you follow God's Divine Truth, remember to look people directly in the eye and speak the emotional truth at all times. Reduce your crow's feet and wrinkles around the eyes by being yourself and processing your emotions as you are being honest. Do not worry about others reactions. Your emotional truth will not only help to detoxify your soul and your body but will also help others deal with their emotions. After all, you are also their Law of Attraction, their messenger of truth, so your interaction with them is helping them to heal their souls. Be a leader of truth and transparency in this new evolutionary, feminine era.

You are an individual soul with an individual mission so follow your desires and inspire others to live their best life. Do not allow anyone to stop you singing the song in your soul and expressing the unique gifts you were born with. Your passions and desires are important to your youthfulness and health so create a job that makes you feel joyful. Your life will be richer in so many ways if you follow your passion instead of just a big pay check.

Set your powerful intention and get ready for increase. Keep believing, keep following God's laws, and keep your heart and mind open for your Law of Attraction to kick in. This is the year to step into the blessings that you have always imagined. Maybe you need a breakthrough in your finances or in a relationship. Whatever you desire, let your dreams be fulfilled by being fueled with the burning passion inside of you and by following the truths of God, not by being competitive or hungry for power. We were never designed to be competitive. We were born to co-create and cooperate. The universe is supremely abundant and full of energy that is ready to support you, so release your fear and fill the lack inside of you with hope.

Finally, avoid all chemicals and addictives. Do not ingest or put anything in your body that you cannot spell or understand. If you cannot eat it, do not put it on your hair or skin. It is most probably toxic, and it will block your pores, cause disease, and age you. Keep your beauty therapy organically pure so your body can become naturally radiant and healthy.

Do not feel discouraged if you do not see overnight changes. You will notice changes to your hair, eyes, or skin in a few weeks. Others may notice you are looking increasingly youthful before you do. But you will see a shift, and you will regain your youthful appearance. As Confucius said, "Everything has beauty, but not everyone sees it." Make sure you see, speak, and live your beauty, light, and truth. Start and end your day by saying, "The Truth will set me free."

## • *Exercises for Eyes, Hair, and Skin* •

### Exercise 1: See the Truth

- Stand in front of the mirror. Move closer. Look deeply into your own eyes. Do not look away. Stare into your soul. What do you see? Do you see the secrets you are hiding? What secrets are you carrying around that you do not want anyone to know?
- Speak the secrets out loud. Release the emotion of guilt, fear, and shame that you are burying inside of you. Keep saying your secrets out loud until there is no emotional charge.

### Exercise 2: Speak the Truth

- Find a close friend or your partner—someone you can trust and confide in. Stand in front of a friend and look into his/her eyes. Try to hold his/her gaze without looking away. Speak out loud the emotions you are feeling as you lock eyes. Are you feeling frightened, shameful, guilty, embarrassed, or upset? Whatever you are feeling, speak it out loud to your friend. Say it out loud again and again until the emotion is clear and you can look into your friend's eyes without a desire to look away.
- Then share a secret with your friend or partner. Bare your soul. Feel and release the fear and shame that comes up from inside of your soul. Feel your friend or partner's reaction. Is he or she judging you? Feel your emotions. Does the person still like you? If he or she does not respond positively, feel your emotional grief. You have triggered something inside that he or she does not want to feel. You are now emotionally free, and your confidant is not. He or she is still carrying things around inside that affect his or her Law of Attraction. You are purifying and living in truth which will positively affect your Law of Attraction.

### Exercise 3: Live in Truth

- Ask yourself the following questions: What am I afraid of? Am I living from my pure soul or from my fear-based personality? Am I living my true passion and desire when I go to work every day? Is the relationship

I am in aligned with Divine Truth and Love, or am I staying because of emotional addiction and fear? Say out loud the truth about your relationship, your career, and other situations in your life. Breathe deeply. Feel and release the emotions that surface. Set about healing all of those false situations in your life.

- Make a list of people in your inner circle. How many people on your list are you not truthful with?
- Now I want you to have an imaginary conversation with the people on your list. What would you say to them? How do they impact your life? If you would still like to keep them in your inner circle, how would you like your relationship with them to change? Process the emotions that come up as you rehearse your conversation out loud.
- Process the emotions of rejection. What if they do not want to talk to you again when you tell them how you feel? Make sure you are emotionally prepared for letting people go before you speak to them.
- Ask the people on your list if you can have a conversation with them. Speak to them about your feelings. Feel and release the emotions that come up as they respond to you.

**Exercise 4: Recognize Your Law of Attraction**

The only way to ensure that you are following the principles of the Laws of Attraction and Cause and Effect is to practice, practice, and practice to reprogram your mind so it accepts that everything playing out around you is due to your soul condition. It is only through processing your emotions and changing your soul condition that you can create a new reality.

- Embrace the fact that everything entering and leaving your life is your own personal Law of Attraction. All the people, places and events in your life are your Law of Attraction.
- Welcome your own Law of Attraction as God's messenger of truth about your soul condition. It shows you what needs healing inside.
- Release any causal emotions in you that may block your Law of Attraction.
- Do not hate, judge, or blame yourself for your own painful Law of Attraction.
- Never blame or get angry with others when painful events happen.

- Trust that as you release your causal emotions your Law of Attraction will positively change.
- Make a list of all the things that happened in your day—the good and the bad. This is your Law of Attraction.
- Turn the radio on. What song is playing? What subject are they talking about? This is your Law of Attraction. You are receiving a message to heal your soul or fulfill your life purpose.
- Did you have an argument today? The person you argued with was your Law of Attraction. What did the person show you that you needed to heal in your soul?
- Why did an angry woman or man attack you? There is something in your soul that attracted their attack. Do you remember feeling like this when you were a child?
- Did you make good money today? Did you struggle to make ends meet? This is your Law of Attraction. What do you need to heal in your soul so you can make money? Do you feel unworthy or that money is bad?
- How is your marriage? Are you single or unhappy in love? This is your personal Law of Attraction. What do you need to heal in your soul to find true love and your soul mate?
- Are you struggling with getting pregnant? This is your Law of Attraction. What is your messenger of truth? What do you need to heal in your soul? Are you fully balanced in your feminine energy or have you chosen a partner who is not ready to be a parent? Both you and your partner need to assess your Law of Attraction. Perhaps your infertility is happening because deep down inside your soul wants to adopt a child in need who has already been born.

**Exercise 5: Recognize That Your Child is Your Law of Attraction**

- When your child is misbehaving or having problems, do not spank or shout at your child. Instead, process your own emotions and Law of Attraction.
- Ask yourself: "What is my child showing me that needs healing in my own soul?" "Where have I felt this emotion before?" "Did I feel like this when I was a child?" When you get the answer, process that emotion out of your soul by feeling and releasing it.

- Begin to honor your child's free will. Process your feelings of control and fear until they have cleared.
- Once again, observe the adults and teachers surrounding your child. They, too, are your own Law of Attraction because your child has no free will. Your child is surrounded by your friends and neighbors or is going to a school that you sent him or her to. Recommend to the adults in your life that they process their unresolved emotional injuries rather than project onto your child. Feel and release your own emotions of fear or embarrassment as you speak out to protect your child.

**Exercise 6: Live Your Passions and Desires**

- Before you can ask God for anything, you must first know what it is that you desire. Most people cannot manifest the life of their dreams because they do not really know what it is that they want. Take time to sit and listen to your inner voice and decide what it is that you really desire to manifest. Release any causal emotions that may cause you to desire something that is out of harmony with God's truth and love.
- List all the things that you loved to do as a child. Did you love to paint, sing, dance, cook, run, tell jokes, or build things? What was your passion? Connect to your original self before the damage, conditions, and belief systems set in and suppressed your dreams.
- Make a collage of pictures from magazines that depict your dream or draw a picture and color it in—with lots of intricate detail. The more you can visually depict and express your passions and desires, the more you can pull down the energy from a mere etheric thought and feeling into physical matter and reality.
- Once you have decided what it is that you really want, you must focus your feelings on it. When you focus on your desires with an immense feeling of love, which is the highest vibration of energy, you then attract them into your life. The more passionate the desire and love for those things that you want to achieve and bring into your life, the more they can materialize.
- You must then believe and feel as if the object of your desire has already arrived. Close your eyes and feel what it is like to have this dream come true. The more you can visualize and feel that your dream has already

happened, the more you can turn it into a physical reality.

- Be open to feeling all of your emotions. Release all the negative emotions in you such as fear, guilt, or shame about fulfilling your Law of Desire. Keep releasing emotional injuries until you feel worthy enough to receive what you desire.
- Pray to God for help. Pray to God to remove the causal emotions in you that block your Law of Attraction.
- Always remember that God is infinitely wiser than you are and what you desire may not necessarily be for your highest good. Now you have made your request, let go and trust. God will send you the best thing for your life.

**Exercise 7: Acupressure for the Eyes**

The following exercise is an excellent massage technique that will help to rid your eyes of crow's feet. Practice it every day and see the results:

- Apply some organic eye cream to your middle fingers. Place them at the inside line of your eyebrows. Apply pressure and move the fingers along the top eyebrow line, pressing as you go.
- Press all the way around the eye, paying particular attention to the crow's feet at the corner of the eyes. Then continue with the massage underneath the eye.
- Place the middle fingers on the top of the cheek bones and up along the inside of the nose until you return back to the starting point at the beginning of the eye brow line. Repeat this exercise thirty times, day and night. The eye cream provides extra moisture and stops soreness while you are applying acupressure.
- After you have finished your acupressure session, you may like to apply some orange extract and lemon juice to your crow's feet. Leave the citrus mixture on the skin for about ten minutes. It will tighten and refresh the skin.

**Exercise 8: Reducing Crows Feet**

- Make sure that you have your eyes checked by an eye doctor every year.

If you do not wear the right prescription eye classes or contacts, you will squint and create wrinkles.

- Regularly exercise your eyes to strengthen your eye muscles. Follow your finger up and down and from side to side. Repeat this exercise for both eyes.

### Exercise 9: To Prevent Discoloration and Bags under Eyes

- Rub on the point outside of your outer nostrils. Gently rubbing releases toxins from the body that can show up as blotches and bags under the eyes.
- Slices of cucumber placed on the eyes also reduce puffiness and dark circles. They contain a large amount of ascorbic acid which decreases water retention and therefore, reduces puffiness from around the eyes.
- If your eyes are dry, use eye drops to keep your eyes moisturized— especially during winter when you have central heating. Make sure the eye drops are preservative free.

### Exercise 10: Eat Spinach and Berries for Healthy Eyes

- **Good Eyesight:** Spinach is a rich source of beta-carotene, lutein, and xanthene—all of which are beneficial for eyesight. Beta-carotene is supplied to the eyes by cooked spinach. It can prevent Vitamin A deficiency disease, itchy eyes, eye ulcers, and dry eyes.
- **Age-related macular degeneration (AMD):** AMD or retinitis pigmentosa is responsible for causing blindness. It is due to the degeneration of lutein and xanthene which form a central part of the retina. Consumption of spinach can result in regaining of the two pigments and effectively preventing AMD.
- **Cataracts:** Lutein and zeaxanthin present in spinach act as strong antioxidants thus preventing the eyes from harsh effects of UV rays that lead to cataracts.
- Eat bilberries and blackcurrants to prevent eye fatigue and night blindness.
- Eat onion to treat and prevent cataracts.

**Exercise 11: Scan Your Food**

- When you go shopping, energetically scan the groceries for their energy frequency as shown in Chapter 1. Remember that everything you consume is comprised either of dense or light frequency energy. Stop counting calories and start scanning the energy fields of food instead.
- Pick the foods that resonate with your frequency. Select foods that hold the highest level of light—foods such as fruits and vegetables that are nearest to sunlight and the earth rather than packaged and synthetically made in a factory.
- Avoid buying foods with ingredients that you do not understand or cannot spell. Remember the motto: "If you cannot spell it, do not put it in your mouth."
- Choose foods with an array of colors that are high in antioxidants.
- Eat super fruits such as blueberries, pomegranate, and acai.
- If you body is overly acidic, eat green alkaline vegetables such as kale, barley grass, broccoli, and green beans to ensure the proper PH balance. Eat fruits such as figs, apples, pears, and peaches. Avoid acid-forming animal products.
- Replace wheat, corn, and rice with high protein ancient grains such as amaranth, kamut, spelt, and quinoa.
- Steam vegetables or eat raw live foods to preserve enzymes and nutrients.
- Blending fruits and vegetables together is a great way to get the right amount of nutrition.
- Eat plenty of turmeric, ginger, basil, and other herbs and spices.

**Exercise 12: Detoxifying Your Body**

- Gently detoxify your liver to clear your skin. Take milk thistle supplements or drink milk thistle tea.
- Eat a daily sprig of parsley to detoxify your kidneys. Eat cilantro to remove the presence of heavy metals, a clove of garlic for killing and expelling parasites, or a few drops of olive leaf extract a day to kill viruses.
- Triphala is a powerful detoxifying agent used in traditional Indian

Ayurvedic medicine. It is an excellent colon cleanser and helps to purify the blood. Take it regularly with your breakfast.

- Minimize deadly nightshade vegetables such as eggplant, potatoes, tomatoes, and bell peppers.
- Eat plenty of fiber and whole-grain foods such as oats and bran.
- Cut down on yeast-filled foods such as white bread.
- Eat fruit or honey, especially Manuka honey, instead of sugar and candies.
- Take a spoonful of apple cider vinegar every day to remove bacteria and if you suffer from acid reflux and need more hydrochloric acid in your stomach. On the other hand, drink half a teaspoon of baking soda in a glass of water if you need to neutralize your acidic stomach.
- Reduce acidity in your body by going vegetarian or minimizing red meat; eat fish, white meats, beans, or nuts.
- Erase or minimize the amount of shellfish in your diet.
- Snack on pumpkin, sunflower seeds, or almonds instead of cookies and sweets.
- Bathe in Epsom salts to draw out toxins.
- Go to an acupuncturist and ask him/her to help you unblock your liver, kidney meridians, and release the energy of anger and fear.
- Book a session with a reflexologist or give yourself a foot massage at home. Release the kidney and liver pressure points on your feet.
- Book an appointment with a holistic dentist who is an expert on the removal of mercury fillings. Ensure your immune system is strong enough before you take mercury out of your mouth. Wear an oxygen mask and do not swallow any mercury during the procedure.
- Keep vaccinations to a necessary minimum. If you do choose to vaccinate your child, avoid overloading your child's body with too many vaccinations at one time.
- Use all-natural toothpaste. Choose toothpaste with baking soda for a natural whitening effect. Eat parsley for fresh breath.
- Use a natural hand sanitizer. Do not use antibacterial hand soap with triclosan.
- Avoid aluminum cookware, foil, and food storage products. Do not cook acidic food in aluminum pots. Buy cast-iron, glass or stainless steel pots and pans.
- Never use a microwave.

**Exercise 13: Replenish Your Body with the Elements**

- Drink a glass of water as soon as you wake up.
- Replenish your body continuously with water—at least eight glasses a day and twelve glasses in the winter. Add liquid minerals to the water to ensure that it is alkaline.
- Fit a filter over the tap or use a water filter jug.
- Buy a specialized alkaline machine to transform your water supply into the highest quality of alkaline water.
- Take a walk everyday to get fifteen minutes of sunlight. If you are in a winter climate, make sure you take a daily dose of Vitamin D.
- Walk in the rain or near water to absorb negative ions.
- Take a revitalizing bath—in warm water, not hot! Himalayan salt baths, Epsom salts, or Dead Sea salts are rejuvenating and help to slough off dry skin.
- Buy a humidifier to add moisture to the air in your home during winter or in summertime if you need to have the air-conditioning on.
- Buy a water fountain for your home to ensure that your space is filled with negative ions.
- Turn off electrical equipment to reduce the amount of free radicals in your home.

**Exercise 14: Omegas, Honey, and Probiotics for Hair, Eyes, and Skin**

- Use omega fatty acids every day, such as fish, flaxseed, borage oil, or flaxseed meal in your cereals, salads, or oatmeal. Omega-3s will keep hair, eyes, and skin healthy.
- Take a high grade probiotic and a spoonful of Manuka honey every day to balance your intestinal flora and keep toxic bacteria at bay. Regularly eat natural Greek yogurt, especially when taking antibiotics.

**Exercise 15: Cleanse Your Skin**

- Use a good body cleanser such as tea tree oil or an olive leaf or coconut oil soap which are powerful natural antibacterial and antifungal agents.
- Apply an organic honey all over your skin once a week, especially to the

rougher areas on your body—knees, elbows, backs of arms, thighs, and buttocks. Leave the honey application on for fifteen minutes. Rinse off in the shower.

- Try massaging a handful of Epsom salts mixed with a tablespoon of bath oil or olive oil, and rub all over your moist skin to exfoliate and soften your skin. Then sponge down.
- Use a natural-hair skin brush to exfoliate your skin every day.

**Exercise 16: A Healthy Shave**

To prevent allergic reactions to shaving, use alternative shaving creams containing natural ingredients that are gentle on the skin. There are many natural products available to buy.

- Always look for natural shaving creams that are free of toxic antibacterial agents. Triclosan is a toxic agent.
- Choose plant-based shaving creams or those which contain essential oils derived from plants.
- For an ultranatural shave, use olive oil as a lubricant.
- Aloe is a great skin soother to use after shaving; it prevents nasty shaving bumps.
- Shaving in the shower can be beneficial. The warm water will soften the hair and make shaving easier on you and your skin.
- Beware of using a dull razor. It can lead to a vast array of problems from razor burn and cuts to an uneven shave. There are many razors to choose from now that are technologically advanced and tell you when it is time to change the blade.
- Exfoliating before shaving will benefit a razor and keep it sharp. Dead skin cells clog and dull the blade which can negatively affect your shave and cause skin irritation.

**Exercise 17: Massage and Moisturize Your Skin**

- After exfoliating your skin, perhaps in the evening before you go to bed, draw a bath. Fill it with natural oils such as Vitamin E, jojoba oil, or coconut oil which are especially healing for the skin or you can add a little baking soda once a week. After your bath, massage in a natural body oil containing borage seed or sandalwood oil or a natural cream from a health food store. Do not rub your skin dry, but rather pat it and do not put anything on your skin that you cannot ingest. If you cannot eat it, do not put it on your body.

### Exercise 18: Naturally Fade Age Spots

- Use the juice of a lemon. Dip a cotton ball in the juice twice a day and rub on the skin where the age spots are. The juice of the lemon will safely remove the upper layer of the skin and will help to lighten the spots. This remedy will take anywhere from six to eight weeks before you start to see the spots fade.
- Rubbing a piece of red onion, apple cider vinegar, or noni juice on age spots will also work.

### Exercise 19: Natural Products

- Use an environmentally friendly dry-cleaner. Take your dry-cleaned clothes out of their bags and hang them by a window to clear fumes before you wear your clothes.
- Try to wear natural materials, such as cotton, against your skin.
- Use natural cotton bed linens.
- Use a natural detergent to wash your clothes as well as the surfaces and carpets in your home.
- Decorate your home with nontoxic paint.

### Exercise 20: Hair Maintenance

- Check your thyroid regularly with a doctor or alternative health practitioner and introduce a natural form of iodine into your diet such as sea vegetables.
- Wash your hair with a sulfate-free shampoo and conditioner that contains biotin, keratin, and natural ingredients so your hair is not stripped of its natural oils.
- Take a biotin supplement. Saw palmetto is also a great hair nutrient.

- Avoid brushing wet hair. If you must comb wet hair, use a very wide-toothed comb. Also avoid brushing hair too frequently as doing so can injure hair and increase loss. Use your fingers to undo tangles, not a comb or brush.
- Avoid rubbing hair vigorously with a towel after washing it. This can also lead to hair breakage. Pat it dry gently instead.
- Regularly massage your hair. Bend over so the blood is directed to your head. Massage your hands gently through your hair. Massage deeply into the scalp, and then gently pull the hair at the roots to strengthen it. Do this every night before you go to bed.
- You can also use peppermint, rosemary, coconut, jojoba, or olive oil once a week to massage the hair and give it extra moisture. Hair-growth oil containing Sunnah Black Seed will also help. Leave the oil on for half an hour before you shower, or for a deeper conditioning, leave it on overnight. Wrap a scarf or plastic wrap around your hair or wear a shower cap so you do not stain your pillow. Your hair may look a little limp for a day, but once you shampoo again, it will regain its fullness and any hair loss will stop.
- Get rid of build up on your hair by mixing ¼ cup of apple cider vinegar with one gallon of distilled water. Wet hair with warm water or shampoo and rinse as usual. Then pour two cups over the scalp and let mixture saturate the hair. Finish with a cold-water rinse.

**Exercise 21: Crystal Healing for Hair, Eyes, and Skin**

- For speaking truth and opening up communication centers, place aquamarine, blue topaz, blue opal, and turquoise on your throat chakra.
- Carry or wear brazilianite and magnetite to bring desires to the surface.
- Amethyst, ruby, and topaz help to fulfill ambitions and promote success.
- For hair loss, carry or wear aragonite, blue opal, or selenite. Also chalcopyrite promotes hair growth.
- For poor eyesight, carry or wear agate, aquamarine, or fire opal. You can also place aventurine, fire agate, or jade on the eyelids.
- For skin disorders and irritations, including dry itchy skin, carry or wear fuchsite, selenite, or quartz crystal. You can also apply an elixir of green moss agate, moonstone, or topaz to the skin or drink an elixir of jade.

# 6
# Spiritual Facelift

*In nature, nothing is perfect and everything is perfect.*
*Trees can be contorted, bent in weird ways,*
*and they're still beautiful.*
**Alice Walker**

Put down that knife; let go and surrender to the Divine! You can lift your face and neck naturally as you learn how to trust in a Higher Power. If you respond to life in a totally different way, you can learn to hold your head up high and elongate your torso. Your posture tells the world a lot about you. When you do not surrender to a Higher Power but hold on too tightly, trying to control your life because of insecurity and a lack of faith, you create tension in your neck and shoulders. You become clenched in the jaw, strained in the eyes, pinched around the mouth, and hunched in the shoulders. This tension causes wrinkles in the neck, chest, and face. When we are fearful and insecure, everything in our body caves in. We no longer embody an open, lifted, relaxed stance. That is why if you surrender to the presence of God and under-stand that you are supported and not alone, you will automatically relax and open your neck, shoulder, and facial muscles. From this state of knowingness, you can move through life in a powerful state of ease and grace.

# Nature Is Your Teacher

If you want to lift your face, neck, and torso naturally, you also need to look for a guide in nature, which is God's most magnificent masterpiece. Nature and animals are our greatest teachers. Watch animals as they move through life and interact. Cats show us how to practice stillness, agility, and gentleness; horses embody beauty and strength, and swans teach us how to be graceful and to elongate the neck. You never see a swan pushing and forcing its way through the water. It swims through life with a graceful ease, surrendering and following the current while allowing itself to be propelled forward. You never see a swan swimming tirelessly upstream against the tide. That is how we are meant to walk through life, not pushing and forcing but surrendering and allowing, not splashing uncontrollably but gliding, fully balanced and supported by the sea of life.

But to be able to learn to swim properly and stay afloat, you must first ensure that your body is strong. This means the chakra system must be perfectly aligned and balanced so that your energy flows properly. Your posture must also be upright which means a good muscle tone. Good posture takes years off your appearance. Like a tree, you need a strong trunk to support your branches so you can grow taller and reach towards the light. But to keep your branches strong you must stay grounded and connect to strong roots that anchor you to the earth. Yoga is a great practice to ensure that everything is perfectly aligned, strong, and balanced. As you do the sacred exercises—stretching, breathing deeply, and opening your chakra energy points—you strengthen, lift your chest, and elongate your body. Yoga also helps you pull energy down from the universe, circulating it down through the head and crown chakra and out through your feet. This is a process of bringing heaven to earth. A trick for good posture is to imagine a thread running up your spine and out the crown of your head, pulling you upward.

There are several other practices that can help you with this work. Pilates can help to strengthen and elongate the body. People doing Pilates exercises say they have seen improvements in range of motion, flexibility, circulation, posture, and abdominal strength—and decreases in back, neck and joint pain. Pilates teaches personal awareness of how you sit or stand and how you move. Tai Chi also improves balance, flexibility, and muscle strength. Tai Chi uses many symbols from nature. It teaches you how to move gracefully with the least resistance. The flow of energy and motion regulates your breathing and keeps your posture soft but strong. Qi Gong is also beneficial for training the body to move gracefully. As a spiritual art, it deepens awareness of self and nature while creating a wonderful feeling of peace and harmony.

A daily schedule of core exercises, such as sit-ups, also trains the muscles in your pelvis, lower back, hips, and abdomen to work in harmony. This leads to better balance and stability, either on the playing field or in daily activities. A tree is only as strong as its trunk and roots. Without a strong trunk, the tree would topple over. Through deep breath work, core exercises for your abdomen, and a dedicated yoga, Pilates, Tai Chi, or Qi Gong practice, everyone can look younger and grow a strong trunk with long, nourished, flexible branches that do not break easily but rather bend with the wind.

## KUNDALINI ENERGY

The process of building a strong center and greater lift is accelerated when you remove your emotional blocks and open up your chakra system. When your blocks are removed, you will eventually release a powerful energy called *kundalini* that is coiled at the base of your spine. The word *kundalini* is derived from a Sanskrit word *kundal* meaning a coil. It is the dormant energy present in a triangular bone called the sacrum. This primordial energy within the human body was considered by the saints and sages to contain the highest esoteric knowledge.

The Latin name *os sacrum* suggests that it is a holy part of the body. Egyptians also felt the sacrum was very mystical, the seat of special power, and it has often been referred to in Vedic and Tantric texts. The ancient Greeks were also aware of this part of the body and attributed it to supernatural abilities. They noted that the sacrum is the last bone to be destroyed when the body is burnt.

Kundalini energy is said to nourish the tree of life within us. It usually begins rising as a result of strengthening the energy system through yoga, meditation, or releasing emotional blocks in the body that have previously repressed energy. An emotional trauma can suddenly release kundalini. When released, the kundalini moves from the sacrum up the spinal column like a pillar of light to your brain and pituitary gland. As the fiery current surges through the body, it activates your DNA, igniting the divine spark or God force.

Throughout history, different symbols have been used to depict kundalini rising. It is often referred to as the "serpent power" because the energy in the sacrum is coiled up like a snake. In the West, the sacrum is symbolized as the Holy Grail, the container of the water of life. The word *sarap/seraphim*, meaning serpent, appears three times in the Torah. Moses saw kundalini in the form of a burning bush. In the Bible, Jesus suggests kundalini awakening by saying, "Just as Moses lifted up the snake in the desert, so the Son of Man must be lifted up." (John 3:14) Moses raised it on a staff, which represents the central support of the human body or the spine. Eve's serpent moved through her spine represented in the Bible by the tree, meaning the tree of life. Christians identified the kundalini as a reflection of the Holy Spirit and worshipped its materialization as tongues of flames over the heads of apostles.

In the Tao, the primordial power is described as that of a mother, a spiritual channel within us which links us with the Divine. In the Holy Koran, Prophet Mohammed talked of the day of resurrection when he says that the "hands will speak."

When kundalini awakening occurs, a flow of energy is experienced, and the various chakras can be felt on the hand and fingers. It also pierces through each of the seven chakras. As I mentioned in Chapter 1, this is why we often hear the number seven mentioned in many spiritual texts. Buddha also described the central channel through which the kundalini ascends. He spoke of the "middle path" to achieve nirvana. Buddhist masters considered that kundalini was one of life's greatest secrets, a path of liberation within every human being. They shared information about kundalini with only a few worthy disciples.

Now you, too, have received this ancient secret. When you release your emotional blocks, you release kundalini energy. When you release kundalini energy, you tap into the fountain of youth. Kundalini cleanses and opens all of your chakras so your energy can flow properly. It also opens your third eye so your psychic abilities can develop and you see the bigger picture. It can cause a tingling sensation and a disruption of the nervous system until the energy is integrated.

Once your kundalini energy is released up the center of your spine, you will feel compelled to alter your posture and your life. When the process of integration is complete, your consciousness will feel expanded and your energy will change to a higher frequency. You will begin to feel a sense of unconditional love and peace. You will also feel the need to keep your body aligned and your life in balance at all times. If you go out of balance physically, emotionally, or mentally, you become so aware that you are out of sync that you have no choice but to return to a state of peace, harmony, grace, and balance. It seems that kundalini rising is like an electric fence that keeps you from going out of your emotional, physical, spiritual, or mental boundaries.

## LETTING GO OF STRESSFUL LIVING

When people are fully connected and their kundalini energy has been activated, they begin to see life in an entirely new way. Not only will they notice that their lives are too cluttered, but they will also realize that the world is operating at a completely unnatural pace.

People are rushing and pushing, ambitiously striving, forcing the flow of life. This causes the body to be strained, especially around the neck and shoulders. When people are aligned with their souls and connected to God, their lives have to change. They cannot help but refine their lives and remove the excess negative baggage that weighs them down. They desire to live life in a gentler, simpler way.

You may find you want to retreat into nature or live a more reclusive life for a while because you crave space and silence. Your inner world will become much more captivating than the outer world that is going on around you. You will realize how aggressive, competitive, and noisy the world can be. Most importantly, you will realize that everything you are striving for in the external world is already inside of you. You will turn your eyes inward and have no desire to waste your energy on anything or anyone who does not feel good or drains your energy field. You will ask yourself the question: "Who or what am I carrying?" and feel a strong desire to let your heavy burdens go.

Letting go is an important part of the healing and purification pro-cess because letting go leads you to your authentic self, your pure soul. Letting go can take the form of releasing emotional addictions, mental debris, physical habits, people, places, material possessions, or even an outcome. It is important to clear your inner and outer home regularly to create a space for the new you.

This process of letting go may feel painful at first, but if you do not release things, situations, or people that are harmful or are holding you back from your higher purpose and own spiritual progression, you will not allow your soul to expand. The more you clear, the more you allow light to enter and fill your soul as well as your physical body.

In Chapter 5, you read briefly about how you may have to let go of certain people in your life who do not serve your higher good or do not want you to speak your emotional truth. As you clear your emotional injuries, you may find yourself having to let go of more people from your life. These will be the people whom you were once co-dependent with and addicted to. Once you have healed your emotional addictions, you will most probably realize that some of your relationships were unhealthy. They were either based on insecurity or happened because you had a childhood feeling of being unloved or unworthy.

As I spoke about in Chapter 5, friends that you have known all of your life may also vanish. They may not want to accept the new you, especially if they are resistant to facing their own fears and doing their own healing. They may feel frightened to make a change; they may mock or become angered by you as you step into your greatness. They may accuse you of thinking you are better than they are or say that you have gotten too big for your shoes. Yes, you have grown too big for your shoes! You have to equip yourself with a new pair to support you through the next stage of your powerful life journey. Your stepping up and stepping out may trigger negative emotional projections from oth-ers as you "dare" to be all that God has created you to be.

If you clear your soul of its emotional injuries and connect further to God and God's Divine Truth, then the words or negative behaviors of others will no longer affect you. Dealing with the emotional process of accepting that some people may not like you is an important part of the souls' journey. If you can continue to be yourself and work through all of your emotions so you no longer care how people feel towards you, you can then follow God's Truth, no matter what the consequences. This will help you live with emotional freedom.

If you find it distressing to let people go, then process your grief and do not get angry. Just simply hold a space for them to return one day. Breaking apart may be only temporary. It depends entirely on whether your friends, associates, or family members find the courage to become emotionally honest and undertake their own inner healing. Be prepared that they may never return, but do not let the fear of losing them and being alone hold you back. Your playing small does not ultimately serve anyone. Fly free and reach the highest place inside of yourself. Then you can show the people you love how they, too, can heal. The shift inside of you will show others how to reclaim their power. When you can step into the place where your greatness is visible because you cannot keep it hidden inside any longer, people will want to be in your presence. It will make them feel good and inspire them to live their highest authentic potential.

Letting go of old material possessions can be emotionally difficult as well. But possessions in your home may no longer suit you anymore once you have done your emotional clearing. Just like people, your possessions also have their own particular energy frequency and that frequency may not be the same as your new, purified energy field. Old belongings represent your old self. Clinging onto possessions stems from an inability to release your grief and let go of the past. As you purge your emotions, so you will find yourself continuously wanting to refine your home and clear out your old things. As you become your authentic self, you will probably find your tastes will change anyway and you will want to fill your home with the exciting energy of new belongings. You will desire that your home becomes a beautiful sacred space filled with the highest of energy frequencies. That is why I recommend you choose just a few of your most favorite mementos and make a sacred memory corner in a room in your house. Or you can place your most special possessions in a decorative box. The rest of your things can be donated to someone who is in need. It is important to let go and clear your grief as you release old memories and possessions. Your denial of grief will block your soul's desire for growth and change. Clinging to the old will stop you from expanding and living in the present moment of your new life.

Likewise, we should let go of any attachments that cause us pain if we cannot have them. We live in a society that is very attached to the material and physical world. People feel like they are going to die if they do not get the car that they want or the mansion they have dreamed of all their life. But the truth is that no one is going to die if he or she does not have these things. What will kill you is your ferocious need for money, power, and control.

When we have feelings of insecurity and fear around money, the first chakra gets blocked, which can lead to illnesses such as bowel cancer. Remember, the first chakra is associated with survival and ties to family, especially the mother. When we struggle with our authentic personal power and feel fearful, we also block our third chakra, the solar plexus, which can lead to ulcers and stomach cancer. Excessive stress also lowers the immune system making us susceptible to a whole array of diseases.

This does not mean you cannot like beautiful things; you can love money, beautiful surroundings, and possessions, but why allow yourself to suffer if you do not get exactly what you want. If you are crying because you cannot own that designer dress or that particular house, then you are far too attached to the material world. You need to release childhood injuries that have made you feel unlovable and unworthy without those things. Try visualizing yourself on your deathbed and ask yourself what is going to be important at that moment. I am sure you are not going to be thinking about a Gucci handbag as you cross over to the Other Side.

As was discussed in Chapter 1, your soul is eternal. When you die, the only thing that is going to matter is the condition and contents of your soul, which will be revealed to you when you see the reflection of your spirit body staring back at you on the Other Side. If while you are alive, you focus solely on your physical body and with accumulating material things, which are only temporary, you are going to be shocked when you see your spirit body after death. Even if you have perfected your face through plastic surgery yet have not cleared your unhealed emotions, by the time of your death your soul condition will have deteriorated and deformed your etheric body. That is why it is so important that while you are living your best life on earth, you spiritually prepare for your death. Learning to let go of attachments is key to your soul's evolution.

As your soul development grows, you will probably let go of your aggressive ambitions, too. People push and strive for power because they want control. Having a desire for a powerful job and high status in society rather than a desire to fulfill your passions and life purpose originates from a lack of self-esteem and a feeling of powerlessness. These, too, are emotional injuries from childhood. When we are emotionally wounded, we need people to treat us with respect and see that we are important. Our insecurity creates a need to prove that everyone else is wrong and we are right. The desire to win drives us to work with a fury every day until we crash at the end of the week with exhaustion. This driving force is also present because we do not trust that God will help us fulfill our passions and desires.

Many people also become addicted to glamour. When people act with pride, criticize, or separate themselves from others, it is a sign that glamour has taken hold. Once people are free of these characteristics, they are free of glamour. When I speak about glamour, I do not mean haute couture or Paris catwalks, although glamour can manifest in the form of materiality. Glamour is when people overidentify with materialism and have an insatiable desire for possessions and/or money. They believe these things make them self-important and better than others. Glamour is an exciting allure that leads them to an unrealistic illusionary state in which they feel that they are special rather than ordinary. Glamour boosts the ego. It causes people to over-romanticize the importance of their possessions and position in their own inner and outer worlds.

Glamour takes the form of many things. There is the glamour of sentiment, which is a pseudolove based on attachment and addiction to loving or being loved or the glamour of devotion referring to people who fanatically follow a cause in an extremist fashion. There is the glamour of the path which refers to the glamour of the spiritual path itself. People feel important and better than others because they feel more "spiritual." They are glamorizing the path rather than healing the cause.

There is the glamour of physical strength—body builders, sports stars, models, and many celebrities identify with the glamour of their looks. Then there is the glamour of being busy, the glamour of personal wisdom, the glamour of popularity, the glamour of a nation, the glamour of self-sacrifice, the glamour of war, the glamour of knowledge, the glamour of world saviors and teachers, the glamour of aloofness, or the glamour of psychic perception. Many psychics glamorize their extrasensory gifts and separate themselves from other people.

It is essential to let go of feelings of glamour because those feelings encourage people to avoid their deeper emotions of unworthiness, self-loathing, and insecurity. An attachment to glamour holds people back from consciously evolving and operating from their souls. The spell of illusion can send lives completely out of control.

Once people have rediscovered life's greatest secret and have fully understood that their riches are inside their soul, their self-esteem improves dramatically and they stop either reaching to the outside for validation or shrinking into the background. Their confidence soars, and their necks, faces, and spirits become lifted. They know who they are and all that they are meant to be, and they are not afraid to show it. They walk tall like a regal king or queen whether they have material things or not. They do not have to identify with anything. They know they are a great soul rather than just a body and an intellectual mind. They are fully awakened, aware of their life purpose and powerful presence in the world. They no longer hunch their shoulders or play small. They do not care what others think of them. They have learned to love themselves, no matter how much they own, how they look, or how anyone else treats them. They do not limit their greatness just to make other people feel more comfortable. They are willing to walk alone, if need be, to fulfill God's divine plan and their highest potential.

Through this process of letting go of emotional, mental, and physical debris, you will save energy and will be able to accomplish much more. When you release those things that no longer serve your life, your whole body will feel lighter; you will create an opening for all things new and allow more time to devote to the real you.

## LEARNING TO SURRENDER

This letting-go process can be deepened when you learn to trust and surrender to God. It means trusting that something bigger is playing out in your life and that if something does not work out, then it was not right for you even if you felt convinced that it was at that time. Rejection is God's protection, so if you lose a job, a best friend, or your home, then your soul is calling for something more to help you evolve to a higher level. Your messenger of truth, your Law of Attraction, is showing you what needs healing. That is why you should trust the higher plan and know that deep down inside there is something much better around the corner coming your way.

Two of the most important lessons that you need to master if you want to walk with wisdom are trust and right timing. Lifting your face, neck, and body is the art of doing and non-doing. This means you have to learn when to take action and when to stay motionless and still. You are a human being, not a human doing, so it is important to allow yourself to just *be* and allow things to flow to you instead of rushing around, trying to control things. Your motto should be: "Let go and allow the flow."

As I explained in Chapter 4, this passive act of non-doing is when you are embodying your feminine energy. Knowing how and when to take action and when you should stay still and wait can take time to master. The art of doing and non-doing, giving and receiving, taking action and staying still can be determined only by a feeling. If you feel angry, fearful, vengeful, or guilty about a situation, then it is better to wait, take a deep breath, and process your emotions rather than proceed based on a knee-jerk reaction or charge into a dangerous situation. But after you have cleared the emotions and sat for a while, it will become clear when the time is right to take action. You will have allowed enough time to pass to gather more information; therefore, you can discern more easily what the appropriate action is.

When you practice the art of doing and non-doing, you are forced to surrender to the flow of life. This letting go of the reins can be very hard for most people. Our fear often drives us to want complete control over every situation in our lives. It also makes us want to control the words, actions, and beliefs of other people. We want them to do exactly what we want them to do. We want them to agree with us, like what we like, and live life exactly as we do. If they go against that, we feel threatened.

When you come to terms with the fact that no matter how much you try to control someone, you are never going to be in charge; you can then start to let go and relax. You cannot control anyone; all you can do is release the causal emotions that created your controlling desires and reactions in the first place. Besides, if we try to control someone else, we are trying to stop his or her free will. If you try to stop another's free will, then you are being unloving and out of harmony with one of God's most important laws. Two important questions to ask are: "*Why* do I want control?" and "*What* is the worst thing that can happen to me if I give up control?"

Another powerful way you can discern the need for stillness or action is by learning to surrender to silence. Being silent is one of the greatest gifts you can give yourself. It is in the silence between the notes that we connect to our inner voice, innate intuition, and find God's wisdom. However, people are so terrified of being alone or silent that they fill their lives with a lot of noise, chatter, activities, and people so they do not have to face the silent truth inside of them or fully feel the unhappiness that is playing out externally in their lives.

The emotional disconnect and clutter in our lives causes us to become stressed. When we block the process of facing our true feelings, the buildup of emotions and negative events causes us to have a feeling of being overwhelmed. Remember that your feelings are your inner spiritual guide, so without them you will become lost. You shout: "I can't cope!" but as you learned in Chapter 3, the truth is that you can cope if you emotionally process and do not avoid the truth inside of you. But to access this truth and inner guidance, you have to stop for a silent moment.

Many people also believe in the power of prayer and so they are constantly talking to God and making requests, but what most people do not do is take the time to be quiet and listen for the answers. If you do not find a moment of silence in your day to just sit and listen, then you will not be able to hear the answers God is trying to give you. The real truth lies in the space and the silence in between our thoughts and actions.

If you can be truthful with your answer and honestly process the fear-based emotions that surface when you think about letting go and about being alone, then you can start to bring more ease back into your life. In these sacred moments of grace you will also be able to feel the presence of God. The more we connect to God, the more we can reach a place of perfected love inside of ourselves and stop harming our bodies.

## LIVING A GOD-DEPENDENT LIFE

Living a life without God makes it harder to emotionally process and clear the soul. You have to rely on yourself and the letting go of negative people and things can feel harder because you will feel totally alone. When you surrender to a power much greater than you that sees and knows all things, it is easier to let go of the reins of your own life. God knows much more than mere mortals can ever see for themselves. That is why it is important to become God dependent instead of self-reliant. This is an important distinction.

While it is impossible to get closer to God without accepting Divine Truth, removing emotional blocks, and following God's universal laws, as you read in Chapter 2, many find God dependence difficult because they do not want to live by someone else's rules. Most spiritual seekers prefer to follow a path of Natural Love rather than follow a Divine Love path because it allows a life of self-reliance. Remember, Natural Love comes from within you and is expressed to others. Divine Love comes from God and enters as well as transforms the soul. On the Natural Love path you can remove blocks, follow any path, and develop the love inside of yourself without having God in your life. Buddhism, the New Age movement, Eastern practices, and other intellectually based spiritual paths teach the Natural Love path. You develop love for yourself and others by having adultlike control over your mind and deliberately changing your thoughts and actions. You believe you are God and you can reach your true God state by following many different paths.

On the Divine Love path you are God reliant. You believe that you are God's son or daughter and that you have an emotional relationship with God. God dependency means you have to shift from your personal truth to God's Truth and follow only one path—God's. The Divine Love path incorporates elements of the Natural Love path but focuses on letting go of the mind and developing a childlike feeling. In this childlike state you can clear emotions from the soul. On the Divine Love path you focus on transforming your soul from human to divine by receiving God's Divine Love. When you are on this path, you can reach a state of perfected love, totally free of suffering in two to three years.

When you rely on yourself instead of depending on God, you try to control the outcome of your life and the lives of other people. You often force yourself to avoid your emotions by changing your mind. This means that it could take hundreds of years to become at-one with God, free from suffering. As you learned in previous chapters, the only way to become the person that you want to be is never to ignore the emotion that you feel at this moment. That is the person you are now. If you tell yourself the story that you want to be something different, you force yourself away from your true emotional condition and break your connection with God.

People who learn to surrender to God feel the Divine intelligently guiding their every move and decision. They do not need to be in charge because they have awoken to the fact that they are *not* in charge. They understand that God is ultimately in charge of their lives and the lives of others, so they surrender. This God-dependent life helps them relax, go with the flow, and keep their eyes focused on their own soul's journey.

We are the co-creators of our lives, but ultimately God is supremely more intelligent and powerful than any of us. God has the reins; loosen your grip so that you can receive God's guidance. Take action, then let go and allow the flow. Tell yourself that you have another advisor, other than your own mind; God is going to be guiding you now.

## DEVELOPING A RELATIONSHIP WITH GOD

But how can you begin to let go of control and live a God-dependent life if you have never felt God's presence or believed in a Higher Power? The first thing to understand is that God has a relationship with you whether or not you feel it. Unfortunately, many people do not feel God's presence because they have disconnected from their feelings. But if you are disconnected from God, you are far from home and your true self. God is your creator, a guiding force to lead you to complete happiness, so without God's presence it is going to be difficult to reach a state of perfected love—a sense of heaven inside yourself.

As explained in Chapter 4, people do not realize that they carry a deep grief inside of themselves because they have lost their connection to God. They do not understand the source of so much of their pain which is the fact that since the time of their incarnation, they have been walking around with a gaping hole inside of themselves that was once filled with the love of God. This is the same deep grief that people feel when they wake up to the fact that they are half of a soul and their soul mate is missing. Until you reunite with your soul mate and with God, you will never feel whole. The longer you reject God, the deeper the grief and loss inside of you will be because your soul already knows that there is a painful void. So reconnecting with God should be the main priority in your life.

If you want to develop a relationship with God, you first need to have a desire to know God and to be aware of God's feelings. But in order for you to feel God, you have to have a longing for God's Truth and to be open to experience all your own emotions. If you are emotionally disconnected, then you will block God's presence in your life.

The first thing you need to know about God is that God is not just an entity, an infinite soul, and Super Being that created all things. God also has different qualities and attributes and a personality, just as your soul has a personality. God is not love as many believe, but love is one of the qualities of God. God contains both masculine and feminine energies, qualities, and principles.

God also contains different types of energy: creative energy which some call spirit, pranic energy to maintain creation, a life-force energy, a governing energy that structures all laws, and the Holy Spirit, which connects God's soul to human souls in a personal relationship.

God longs to have a personal relationship with you, but many people often feel uncomfortable with thinking that God has a personality. They cannot even say the word God because it brings up so many negative

## The God Connection

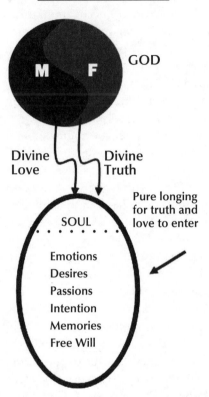

God desires to have a personal relationship with all souls. The removal of emotional blocks allows the soul to expand and connect to God and allows for Divine Truth to enter. The energy of Divine Love is a gift from God. It enters the soul through a connecting pipeline or channel. It is our pure longing that causes Divine Love to enter. Divine Love purifies and cleanses the soul of emotional errors. The soul eventually transforms from human into divine.

emotions inside of them. They objectify God by using a term such as the "Universe" or the "Source."

It is a true fact that God's energy is part of the universe and God's qualities and personality are reflected in the universe, but the universe is only three to fifteen billion years old and God is infinite, so it makes sense that God existed long before the universe was ever created. Describing God as the "Universe" helps people to keep a safe distance from God and remain emotionally disconnected from their true feelings about God.

Then there are those who do not develop a personal relationship because they believe that they actually are God. They focus on developing the "God" inside of themselves. Others believe that yes, indeed, God has both masculine and feminine qualities and principles because they see God's reflection in both men and women and in the whole of nature and the animal kingdom, but they also believe that there are many gods for many different characteristics. Then there are those who strongly disagree with God being one entity because even though they have been taught that God is an entity, they have also been taught that God is but one part of three entities. The idea that one entity created the whole entire universe is hard for many people to believe because of the scale of the creation and their ingrained beliefs. Some people do believe that there is only one God, but that he is definitely not also a "she" and that "he" demands constant worship and attention. Others believe that God is an entity, but an entity who will only love them when they are good and will send them to eternal hell when they are bad. The problem with all of these beliefs is that none of them are true.

Our relationship with God is not only damaged by false societal and religious beliefs but also by our relationship with our parents. Our relationship with God is directly reflected in our relationship with our parents. If one of our parents was absent, then we may have issues around the masculine side of God (the Father) or the feminine side of God (the Mother) and feel that God does not exist at all. Or we may be angry with God and feel as if we have been abandoned. If either parent was abusive, then we also may feel that God is violent and cruel. Then there are those who feel unworthy of God's love. They believe God's love is conditional; they believe all are sinners without fully understanding the true meaning of sin. They feel they can never be perfect enough to be loved. They have been taught that God is wrathful, punishing, and unforgiving. They fear God and think he damns for all eternity. Because of this, they feel judged and unloved just as they have been judged by their parents so they reject God's presence in their lives.

Many God-loving homosexuals have abandoned their belief in God altogether because they have been so mistakenly condemned and taught that God feels they are sinful and evil. Many homosexuals have turned to drugs instead because the pain of the loss of God is so unbearable. They abuse themselves because of a lack of self-love. People from all walks of life turn to drugs—not only as a way to numb their feelings from the pain they feel inside but also because they want to recapture the "high" of the God connection. They desperately try to open a doorway to the spiritual world. That is why drug and alcohol programs which connect addicts to a Higher Power and a spiritual path are so successful.

The instinctual desire for God is there inside all of us, but our trust in God has been broken over and over again by false societal beliefs and by our parents when they broke our trust and loved us only conditionally.

The truth is God does not have a punishing, conditional, or judgmental personality. God is unconditionally loving, compassionate, wise, and merciful. God sees us all as perfect, and God does not judge. God forgives instantly and at all times, no matter what we have done. God has no demands or expectations and expects nothing in return, even though God does long for us to have a relationship if we so desire. God always respects our free will. In fact, God believes that the Law of Free Will is one of the most important laws—even if your free will takes you down the wrong path. Every person has the right to do whatever he or she chooses despite the consequences for his or her soul. Remember, God's laws were not created to punish but to lovingly bring us back into harmony, to a place of perfected love. God's universal laws are a perfect example of how God loves. You will read more about God's love and how it can teach us to love in Chapter 7.

In today's busy world, there are many distractions that interfere with our relationship with God, but as I have emphasized, our desire for God should be our primary focus in life. God put a divine spark in our soul so we would instinctively want to wake up to the truth of who we are and return to being at one with God. Despite this spark, many people remain distant and self-reliant rather than God dependent. They do not trust that God will take care of their needs. This false belief about God, once again, stems from many parents not taking proper care of their children's emotional, spiritual, and physical needs.

Healing your negative beliefs and emotions around God will keep your body relaxed, healthy, and youthful. If you become God dependent and put your relationship with God first in your life at all times, you will completely lift the stress from your shoulders and return to a place of peace and joy. When you keep God in first place, great changes will follow. When you allow God, your divine Mother and Father, to take care of you the way you have never been taken care of before, you will connect to your childlike spirit again and find miracles happening in your life. As you unload your burdens to God, you will always be rewarded because when you trust and surrender to God; you allow yourself to fully receive.

Your childlike feeling of trust will help you run free in life. You can rest in God's loving arms and know that your worries will be taken care of as long as you stay in a place of emotional honesty. You will no longer have the fear or the stress that things will not work out. This means you will not project fear-based energy into the universe, and so you will not negatively impact your Law of Attraction. Yet trusting does not mean you do not take action; you have to take action, but the action you take happens only because you are emotionally honest. If you lie to yourself about the true reason for your action or your desire, then it will only result in harm to yourself.

If you are in conflict with someone, you can place him or her in God's hands, too, and ask God to take care of you both instead of depleting your energy and fighting to prove who is right or who is wrong. As long as you are emotionally truthful about your real feelings and stop focusing on the other person, then all will be resolved. You will be able to ultimately resolve the conflict inside of you that is reflected in your disagreement with another person. God's laws of Natural and Divine Love will take care of bringing harmony back into both of your individual lives. But you will continue to be in discord if you lie to God about why you are fighting with someone else and try to avoid your own Law of Attraction and negative emotions.

## GETTING PERSONAL WITH GOD

It will not be hard to put God first once you get to know God. God is actually your true Mother and Father. This may feel strange, but if you can embrace this truth and understand the real relationship you have with your physical parents, then you will be able to heal your relationship with them and have open and honest communication. You will understand that in the eyes of God your parents are also God's children, which makes them your brother and sister. They were your guardians when you were young and they gave you physical life, but you were created first by God, as were they. Your parents do not own you but are equal with you in the eyes of God. Likewise, when you understand that your parents are also children of God, you can look at them with eyes anew and not label them or project anger on them but see them as souls, trying to evolve just as you. If you and your family can embrace this Divine Truth and treat each other as brothers and sisters, understanding that you have the same divine parent, then your relationship can become equal, harmonious, loving, and truthful.

God is not just your true parent; God really is the most wonderful friend you will ever have even if you do not yet realize it. Building a relationship with God is just like building a relationship with any other person. When we first meet someone we like, we have a burning desire to know all about them—the good and the bad, the past mistakes, the future desires. We want to know what they feel about so many things. As two friends open up to one another and start to share and exchange their real feelings, love starts to flow between them. This is how you build a relationship with God.

But the wonderful thing is that you do not have to go through the awkward "getting-to-know-you" process because God already loves you and knows all about you. God has great insight into your soul and knows every causal emotion and every desire that causes you harm and damages other people. You will not have a better friend in your life with whom you can totally be yourself all the time. But if you project a false image of yourself and lie about how you feel, then you will block God's relationship and stop God from helping you.

The problem is that so many people feel they have been let down by love that they dare not trust God. They cannot be truthful about who they really are or how they really feel inside for fear that they will be abandoned or punished, just as their parents judged and punished them. They find the concept of someone loving them unconditionally such an alien experience that it is hard to accept that someone would love and forgive them, no matter what.

The only time they seem to reach out is when things are going wrong and then they have a tendency to blame God for their problems. This gives them an excuse for turning their back on God so they can avoid their own emotions and not take responsibility for their own Law of Attraction. But God did not create any of man's harmful actions or the pain that he or she feels in his or her life. God created only the potential for disharmonious behaviors by creating the Law of Free Will. But to blame God for man's destructive words and deeds is an excuse and an avoidance of emotional truth. Do not waste your time and energy blaming God for the state of the world. God is constantly trying to bring man back into balance through the love of God's divine universal laws.

So learn to prioritize your life and develop a burning desire for God. Make your relationship with God the first priority. Next, give your love to your soul mate, and then you can turn your attention to other people, events, or things. If you live life in that order, then all your needs will be taken care of, and you will find your life will be full of love, support, and abundance.

Start talking to God today. Even if the first conversation you have with God is: "I do not know who you are." "I do not even know if you exist." "I feel like you abandoned me." "I do not know if I like you." Ask God to help you develop a desire to be closer and commit to being emotionally honest. Learn to talk to God every day about how you are feeling. As you develop a burning desire for a relationship and a longing to receive God's Love, you will start to relax into a childlike state. You will start to enjoy being known for who you really are. Your life will change and your relationship with your friends and family members will also transform because you will have someone else to turn to. You will no longer project your emotional injuries onto them even if they are the root cause.

# RECEIVING GOD'S DIVINE LOVE

One of the most powerful laws and gifts from God to help you clear emotional injuries is the Law of Divine Love. Divine Love is as powerful a gift as the Law of Free Will because it transforms your soul. Divine Love is an emotion (energy in motion) from God. It is a substance that can flow from God into your soul through a channel or pipeline called the Holy Spirit, just as the love of another human being can flow into you. But this kind of love differs from the natural love that humans are born with. Divine Love belongs to or is part of God. The Holy Spirit is the connection via which your soul is joined with God's soul. It allows the flow of God's Divine Love into your own soul when you long for it. Divine Love can literally transform your soul from the human to the Divine and assist you in becoming an immortal spiritual being. It enables you to embody the divine nature of God.

God's Divine Love is waiting to be given freely to everyone who asks. But it cannot enter you unless you have a desire for it to flow into your soul. God will never interfere with your free will. It is a matter of knowing in the first place that Divine Love exists, and that it is your will and your desire to possess it that will cause it to flow as a gift into your soul. But Divine Love cannot enter if you are not willing to heal all of your emotional injuries. If you are willing, God's Divine Love can accelerate your emotional release process by helping to remove the blocks. As the Divine Love takes possession of the soul, all the emotional penalties and errors disappear. But if you are not emotionally honest, then the connection with God will break and the flow of Divine Love will stop. The Holy Spirit cannot maintain a connection with the soul when your soul is in an untruthful condition. If you choose to lie or withhold the truth about your passions, desires, longings, and feelings—even to yourself—then the connection with the Holy Spirit is automatically broken. You will be unable to receive any more Divine Love until you reestablish the connection by once again living in emotional truth.

This is the only way you can achieve this divine state. You cannot be "saved" or become "born again" by mere words or through the actions of another human being. No one can feel and release all your negative emotions for you. Only you can heal and transform your soul with

God's assistance. It takes time to release all of the emotions that are frozen in your soul and to purify your soul with the inflow of Divine Love. It does not happen in an instant as many have been taught.

If you start to incorporate a longing for God's Divine Love in your daily prayer practice and believe with all sincerity that this Divine Love will be gifted to you, you will begin to feel this influx of love entering and cleansing your soul. It will feel so incredible and real to you that your belief in a higher, more powerful force will never waiver.

## DEVELOPING YOUR FAITH

***Faith is taking the first step before you've seen the whole staircase.***
**Dr. Martin Luther King, Jr.**

If you want to develop in love and learn to surrender your life to a higher power, it is important to develop your faith. But what is faith and how does it change the way a person lives his or her life? Faith is the confident belief or trust in a person, concept, or thing. Faith is when you have an assured expectation of the things you hope for. It helps you determine truth and helps you act upon the truth.

In today's world, many people are skeptical of the whole idea of faith, because they feel it is something not connected with the ordinary processes of the mind. When you have faith, you believe deep down in your heart and you accept something that your intellect sometimes struggles to accept. Many believe that faith is actually opposed to the convictions of the intellect. Since faith implies a trusting reliance upon future events or outcomes, some people take it as synonymous with a belief not reliant on logical proof or material evidence. But there is always evidence to accompany faith and an evident demonstration of reality, though often it is unseen. You realize this by looking at all the things that happen in your daily life. Every day you believe that the sun is going to come up in the morning and the moon is going to put you to bed at night. You believe these things even though the force that gets the sun to rise and set is invisible. So if you hear anyone say that they believe only in things they can see, then you know that they are lying. They are lying because they believe that gravity will enable them to walk on the planet and stop them from floating off into space every day, and they believe this even though the force of gravity is invisible.

There are many things in our daily life that we trust without seeing. You cannot actually see the wind with your eyes, but there is evidence that it exists. You can feel it on your face and hair or hear it rustling in the leaves. You cannot see it, but you can feel it—you know it exists. This is faith. Faith always has proof even if the proof is just a feeling. There is no such thing as blind faith. The faith is there because the evidence is there.

We can focus this same faith towards God by looking at the evidence. But to do this we need to separate the world that man has created from the world that God created. If you turn to nature, you can see life, nourishment, support, and comfort. The krill in the sea feed the bigger fish that help feed the sea birds and sea mammals. By looking at nature we can see that every component of the ecological system works together to support one another: from a tree giving shelter or providing fuel to a bee pollinating the plants so they will grow, multiply, and blossom or a simple fly playing an important role by eating bacteria. From the smallest seed to the largest mammal, every part of the ecological system plays an important role and is interdependent.

From looking at nature and how all the elements symbiotically work together, we understand that there must be a designer to these glorious workings. If nature thinks, feels, and functions for itself, then there must have been a designer, just as there was a designer for your car or your washing machine. If you want to learn to drive your car properly, you need to read the manual before you use it. So why, if you want to know more about yourself and the world around you, do you not speak directly to the Creator who designed you?

Nature is all the proof we need to see that God exists and to show us that God is a loving force interested in cooperation, abundance, and harmony. Unfortunately, man has taken over the planet, and instead of continuing to develop this cooperative system that provides for every animal and human, he has put in place a system of greed and competition. The planet has changed from an abundant garden that feeds and provides for all of God's children to a place that is full of lack and suffering. The planet is dying; some breeds of animals are becoming extinct; wars are being fought all over the world as men fight against men to dominate and control the natural resources. Meanwhile, the food source and water supply are becoming more and more scarce because of man's competitive nature and addiction to overconsumption. The planet is a reflection of the internal emotional injuries of humans. The world today is not the planet that God created.

Do not allow the painful scenarios and images that fill your television screen on a daily basis lead you to believe that God does not exist or wishes to punish and harm you. As Albert Einstein concluded, "God is subtle, but he is not malicious." Look to nature and have faith that God is good, that God exists and loves you and wants to provide for you. But make sure that when you have faith, you also take action. Faith without action is irrelevant. You cannot experience faith just by sitting there and understanding it intellectually—you need to put it into action and do something to prove that faith exists. It is only by our doing that we practice faith.

Follow the example of past inventors such as the Wright brothers. They had faith that their technical machine could fly before they even proved it could. They had faith because they had seen a bird fly and they believed that they could create a flying machine just like a bird. If they had not had faith, none of us would be flying in the skies today. If you do not develop your faith, you may find that the same happens to you.

So take that first step in your life even though you cannot see the staircase that Dr. Martin Luther King spoke about. If you keep your faith, your stairway to heaven may not feel like climbing a high mountain. Your next step maybe the only step you need to take to reach the summit of your dreams.

Even if things take a long time to arrive, do not give up. Even if negative things have happened, keep going. Many times our dreams do not come to fruition because we get discouraged and give up too soon. You need to develop an unshakable confidence and believe that God will never let you down. Stop focusing on the goal; instead, focus on each individual moment of the journey. Do not get caught up in instant gratification. Just because it does not happen our way on our timetable does not mean it is not going to happen. Every story has a happy ending so if it is not happy, then it is not the end. God's last chapter for you will never end in a negative. God will always make sure you will be at the right place at the right time. If you delay the gratification, the reward will probably be even greater. Just like a bank account, your good karma will accumulate interest and you will be showered with riches at the perfect time. God will never fail you. God can never break a promise because it goes against God's nature. So do not let people talk you out of your dreams because of their fear and lack of faith. Do not get discouraged if you have debt, ill health, a broken relationship, a home foreclosure, or you did not get that job you wanted. God will always make your dream come to pass, even if it looks impossible and illogical. God will pay you back for unfair situations, and if you dare to trust God, the secret desires in your heart will come to pass.

## DEVELOPING A PRAYER PRACTICE

One of the most powerful ways that you can develop your relationship with God, remove your emotional blocks, and have your passions and desires fulfilled is to develop a devoted prayer practice. You can build a strong relationship with God through prayer. You can also receive God's Divine Love through praying; anything your heart desires can be yours as long as it is in alignment with God's laws.

The most important way to develop a prayer practice is to remember the power of your emotions. Prayer is an emotional exchange with God. It is the feeling and the heartfelt desire that activates a response. It is not an intellectual thought, word, or belief. Neither is prayer a demand of God or an expectation that God takes responsibility for our own decisions and actions.

Remember, emotions are the seat of your soul, and it is a soul-to-soul connection that you want to create with God. The more feeling you can put into your prayers, the more powerful the effect. If you pray with earnestness and a passionate longing, then your desire will be felt and God will answer. This is why it is so important to create an emotional relationship with God and see God as an emotional being rather than an inanimate object. The more you can connect emotionally, the more you will feel a response. If you believe that God is merely an electrical power plant that supplies energy instead of a living entity, the infinite soul, and your divine parent, then you will not be able to have a personal relationship with God. You will not be able to feel passionately or connect emotionally. Likewise if you pray to the universe instead of praying to God who created the universe, then the power of your prayer will be diluted. If you deny an emotional connection with God, it will be harder to get your prayer answered.

As I spoke about earlier in this chapter, this inability to emotionally connect with God or even say God's name comes from a childhood emotional injury stemming from our relationship with our own parents and the many false belief systems that have been told to you about God. So keep focused on healing your relationship with God while you are developing your prayer practice.

Even if you do have an emotional relationship with God and pray for more money or a nice house, that prayer will not necessarily achieve the response you want. As I discussed in Chapter 5 about the Law of Attraction, if you have an emotional block such as unworthiness and deep down you do not believe you deserve a new car or you want a car because you want to feel better about yourself, then your prayer will not be answered.

God will never assist in the avoidance of our emotions; that would be unloving. That is why when you pray, it is more effective to pray to God to ask to remove any emotional blocks that are stopping you from creating abundance or buying that new house or car. Pray to have the causal emotion removed that made you feel insecure when you were a child rather than praying for the house itself.

If you pray to God with a feeling and a longing for God to remove your causal emotions so you can achieve your passions and desires, then you will start to see triggers appear in your life. These emotional triggers will appear through your Law of Attraction. Different people and events will show up to push your buttons. Their interactions with you will show you what needs clearing in you. They will help you release the blocks inside of your soul that are stopping you from fulfilling your heart's desires. If you pray at night before you go to sleep, you may have vivid dreams that play out scenarios to trigger a certain emotion in you. If that happens, then it is important to process how the dreams made you feel so you can release your causal emotional block rather than focus on the story and the events happening in the dreams. Remember, the sooner you can clear a feeling, the sooner your soul will purify and your prayers will be answered.

You can pray for all sorts of things to help your life. You can pray for God to show you what emotion is stopping you from opening up to love and a new partner or to show you what emotion is causing the same negative Law of Attraction with a person over again or why you cannot find forgiveness for a loved one. You can pray to remove all sorts of blockages from your soul. You can also pray for God's Truth to be revealed to you, and most importantly, you can pray for God's Divine Love to purify your soul. You will begin to receive all of God's gifts as your daily prayer practice strengthens.

So say your prayers morning and night; open your heart to God, and have a passionate desire for a connection, stay open to feeling all of your emotions. The soul who prays passionately will never be ignored.

## CONCLUSION

Now that you have been given the inner tools to uplift your face and neck and live your best life, you can focus on diminishing the physical damage you have already done to your body. You will find an array of facial and neck exercises at the end of this chapter. You can do these exercises while sitting at your desk, in bed, or on your sofa.

These exercises will help to firm up sagging cheeks, jowls, and eye muscles and prevent a double chin, loose skin in the neck and throat area. Loose, aging skin is the result of a loss of energy taking place within your skin cells. Your cells have no energy to produce the structural proteins and fatty acids needed to support a firm complexion. This is why nutrients for sagging skin are so important.

It is the neck and throat area that tells the truth about a person's age and about his or her life story. Some people think that a double chin is simply excess weight, but in reality it is the result of terrible muscle tone caused by a lack of self-love. Physical fitness and exercise routines are energizing. Regular exercising once a day of the neck and facial muscles can soon remove excess and give your neck and face a tremendous lift. Plenty of moisture to the skin in the neck area will also ensure you maintain a soft, graceful swan-like neck.

With a long neck and body you can walk effortlessly with grace, ease, and wisdom. You can let God take over and allow positive energy to flow into your life and elegantly glide through your weekly schedule. If you find yourself hustling and bustling to make long-sought dreams come true, take a time out in Mother Nature to really commune with the earth, trees, and sky.

Do not swim upstream, live like a swan and allow your life to unfold and take you where it is meant to go. Practice stillness like a cat and gift yourself a moment of quiet so you can receive guidance. Let go of all negative people, possessions, and distractions. As you take action to fulfill your dreams, have faith that you will get the payoff or payback you deserve through the natural laws and cycles of accountability, reward, truth, and consequences.

God is working every day on a divine plan for you from behind the scenes. Just show up with a childlike spirit and do your best but do not try to control the result. This will help you not be so disappointed if something does not work out as you thought. Remember your motto: "rejection is God's protection."

One of the ways to know the divine plan of God is by opened and closed doors. Often this is how God gets us to do things: by closing some doors and opening others. Are you still knocking on a door that is meant to stay closed for your own protection or are you walking through a side door, the door that God has magically opened for you? If you have just applied for a job and done your best in that interview, stop worrying about whether or not you have got the job. If it is meant to be yours, it will happen. Let go of your stress, detach from the outcome, and let God take care of that open or closed doorway.

When the blessings do finally start pouring into your life, remember to celebrate. Do not apologize or downplay what God has done for you. Be an example of God's goodness so others can see that they, too, can receive great gifts if they live an emotionally honest, God-dependent life.

This is your moment; this is your season. This is your time to believe again. Lift your face, your neck, and your head up high. Walk tall towards the light. Trust that God is opening every door until you are living your very best life.

## • *Exercises for a Spiritual Facelift* •

### Exercise 1: Releasing Activities That Weigh You Down

- Make a list of everything that you do each day of the week.
- Read your list and determine which things make you feel happy, re-energized, and make your load feel lighter. Then determine what feels like a burden and what drags you down.
- Release those activities that do not serve you, drag you down, or keep you from living an emotionally present, soul-based life.
- Release your sense of loss and any fear-based emotions about what others may feel about your decisions to potentially let them down as you reprioritize your schedule.

### Exercise 2: Release People That Weigh You Down

- Make a list of all of the people in your life. Do these people make you feel happy and revitalize your energy or are you co-dependent and addicted to them? Now you are releasing your causal emotions, how many people on your list are purely accommodating your emotional addictions and injuries? How many people on your list weigh you down and are holding you back from your higher purpose?
- Once you have determined who is supportive of the new you, put those names together on a separate list. You are left with a list of all of those people whom you would like to potentially release from your life.
- Practice having a conversation with people on your own first. Process your emotions of fear, shame, and embarrassment. Then share with them how you feel about your relationship and how you would like relationship to change. Do not project anger onto them. Dependent on their response, feel and release the emotions of loss, fear, shame, embarrassment, and grief if you both decide to separate. Remember, the separation does not have to be permanent.

### Exercise 3: Lightening Your Home

- Refine your life regularly. Clear your home and closets of all those possessions that are no longer part of your present life. Put the special mementos that you want to keep but no longer use in a box or create a sacred space in your home as a memory corner to display the most special parts of your life. Then release those possessions that no longer serve or fit with the new you. Give them to someone less fortunate. When you clear an energetic space, then new things can come into your life.

## Exercise 4: Building an Emotional Relationship with God

- Write a letter telling God exactly how you feel about your relationship. Do you love God or do you feel that God regularly abandons you? Do you not even believe that God exists?
- Then start a dialogue with God out loud. Do it even if your relationship begins with: "I don't know who you are or what you are in my life." "I feel like you abandoned me." or "I don't like you." The more you dialogue, the more you will start to heal and feel a presence.
- Write to both the feminine aspect of God—Mother God and Father masculine God. How do you feel about both of them? Write your feelings out on the page.
- Read your list and compare how similar your relationship with God is to your relationship with your parents. Your relationship with God is directly reflected by how you feel about your mother and father. The feminine aspect represents your mother and the masculine aspect represents your relationship with your father.
- Release any emotions of anger, grief, or fear. As you heal your relationship with God, so your relationship with your parents will heal and vice versa.

## Exercise 5: Becoming God Dependent

- Pray to God every morning and every night. Ask that God may strengthen and deepen your ability to surrender. See yourself placing your burdens into God's hands. Feel God's arms around you. Allow yourself to "be like a child." Feel supported.
- Practice giving up the reins. Take the necessary daily actions; then let go

and learn to trust God. You will feel out of control at first but keep handing over your problems to God and processing your fear of letting go. Watch how God works and how powerful and quick the miracles are.

- If you are in dispute with someone, visualize a large hand and place the person you are arguing with in God's hands so you do not have to focus on him or her. Let go of the person and the desire to fight. Focus on releasing your own causal emotions that attracted in this conflict to your life.

## Exercise 6: Developing Faith

- Ask that God strengthen and deepen your faith. At first you may feel that your faith is not developing; give it time and you will soon learn to trust God. If you feel your faith is dwindling, ask God to show you a sign. Watch how in the coming days some small miracle or sign will reassure you that God is working behind the scenes to help you.

## Exercise 7: Developing a Prayer Practice

Pray to God whenever you desire a soul-to-soul communication. Prayers will help you draw in loving relationships and more prosperity as they also help you develop your faith. Remember that the more you can feel and express your desire for God's Love and assistance, the more your prayers will be answered.

- Pray morning and night. Focus on your heart area when you pray. Feel your desire for God's help; do not intellectualize your prayer. Passionately say your prayer out loud. Feel the longing. The more heartfelt your prayer, the quicker you will progress and the more you will receive.
- Ask God to help you feel all of your causal emotions.
- Ask God to help you release all of your causal emotions.
- Ask God to reveal your emotional injuries through your Law of Attraction.
- Ask God to remove the causal emotions that block you from your soul mate.
- Ask God to remove the causal emotions that block you from abundance, health, and love.

- Ask God to help you to find the courage to fulfil your passions and desires.
- If your faith is failing, ask God to send you a sign to show you that your dreams are still in motion.
- Ask God to help you develop your faith.
- Ask God to help you trust in God's divine plan for you.
- Ask God to purify your soul by filling it with Divine Love.

## Exercise 8: Aum or Om for Kundalini Rising

In Hindu tradition, *Aum,* also spelled *Om,* is the purest name of God. It is the sound of the supreme consciousness. When you repeat Om, Hindus feel you actually take the name of God. The chanting of Om or Aum purifies the atmosphere and the vibrations of Aum stimulate your root chakra and kundalini rising. Practice the following chant or meditation. Remember to only use this exercise as a form of support to your emotional process. It is the removal of emotional blocks that will release kundalini from your sacrum. It is the feeling and desire of your heart that will connect you to God. In addition to doing this meditation, make sure you speak to God every day and pray with your heart, rather than try to spiritually intellectualize with your mind.

- Sit in a comfortable, undisturbed place. Take a deep breath. Chant Om or Aum at least seven times in succession. Allow the sound of Aum to resonate in the back of your throat and travel from your root chakra up your spine. Make each breath last as long as possible. Take a deep breath and chant again. After seven Aums, stop chanting and sit for a moment of silence. You will feel a sense of peace.

## Exercise 9: Connect Your Child to God

- Encourage—do not force—your children to build a close relationship with God. Encourage them to talk to God as well as you every day, especially if they ever have a problem. This should be easy as children are often very God focused.
- Explain that you are your children's protector and physical guardian, but

God is their divine parent. Teach your children about their own incarnation and reason for life. Explain that you are both children of God. Process your own controlling emotions.
- Show your children how to pray with a passionate desire from their heart.

**Exercise 10: Toning the Face**

- This exercise will help tighten sagging jowls and pouches. Place your fingertips right on top of the lines running from the corner of your outer nostrils down to the corners of your mouth then smile widely. Apply enough pressure on these folds as you smile with your teeth bared. This is a resistance exercise so you must not let go of the pressure while smiling. Press your fingertips down for about five seconds, and then release the resistance. Repeat thirty times.
- This exercise is good for firming and toning the cheeks, jowls, chin, and neck. Look at the ceiling by tilting your head backward. Press your tongue to the roof of your mouth and swallow. Then bend your head slightly to the left and swallow. Bend your head to your right and swallow. Your tongue must be touching the roof of your mouth throughout the exercise. Repeat four times in all three directions.
- Tighten your sagging eye muscles and lift the brow area with this very simple exercise. While keeping the brow relaxed and unruffled, widen your eyes as you would in a state of shock or surprise. Focus looking straight at one point for ten seconds. Repeat this exercise four more times.

**Exercise 11: Toning the Neck and Throat**

Do these firming neck and throat exercises every day, and you will see great results.

- Sit down with your legs folded in comfortable position. Keep your spine straight and tilt your head behind slowly. Hold for ten counts and feel the stretch under the jaw line. Tilt your head back straight and repeat for five sets.
- Sit upright. Lift your head back so you are looking at the ceiling. Keep your lips closed and start a chewing movement. You will feel the muscles

working in your neck. Repeat twenty times.
- Sit upright. Lift your head back so you are looking at the ceiling. Keep your lips closed and pucker them until you are doing a kissing motion. Extend the kiss as if you are trying to kiss the ceiling. You will feel the muscles working in your neck. Repeat ten times.
- Sit upright. Lift your head back so you are looking at the ceiling. Move your mouth wide open as if you are smiling and clenching your teeth and then move your mouth wide open from top to bottom as if you are stretching your upper lip down. Alternate these two movements twenty times.
- This exercise can be done in a seated or standing position. Pull your spine straight up and leading with the chin, gently rotate your head from one shoulder to another. Work your way to doing full head rolls. If full circular motions hurt your neck, you can do semicircular motions instead. Do a full roll three to five times.
- Remember to moisturize your neck and not just your face. Massage natural cream or oil all over the neck with upwards strokes.

## Exercise 12: Elongating the Body Temple

- Find a qualified yoga or Pilate's instructor in your local area or buy a DVD to follow at home if you feel confident in doing the exercises alone.
- Pilates is great for strengthening your core abs and lengthening limbs. Yoga is also the perfect exercise practice to strengthen your core, lift your body, and open your chakras. Examples of yoga poses for strength and flexibility include:

**The Mountain Pose** to improve posture, balance, and self-awareness.

**The Downward Facing Dog** to build strength, flexibility, and awareness.

**The Triangle Exercise** to stretch the spine, open the body, and help you focus.

**The Warrior II** to strengthen legs and arms, improve balance and concentration, and build confidence.

- Remember to begin your workout regime at a gentle level and work up to a more advanced stage. Breathe deeply through each set of exercises. This will allow you to strengthen and elongate at a deeper level.

## Exercise 13: Strengthening the Core

- Any exercise that uses the trunk of your body without support counts as a core exercise. Abdominal crunches are a classic core exercise. Try lying on your back and placing your feet on a wall so that your knees and hips are bent at ninety degree angles. Tighten your abdominal muscles, and then raise your head and shoulders off the floor.
- Classic pushups count, too. You can also do pushups on your knees or standing up against a wall.

## Exercise 14: Learning to Move Gracefully

- Tai Chi and Qi Gong train the body to move gently and gracefully. Buy a reputable Tai Chi or Qi Gong DVD and practice at home or join a local class in your community.

## Exercise 15: Sitting, Standing, and Walking with Grace

- Hold your back and neck straight when you are sitting, either watching television or working at your computer. Elevate your computer screen so you do not look down and crease your neck muscles. Keep your shoulders back and down and your feet uncrossed. Feel the space between your shoulders and head. Feel your neck stretching. Place your feet squarely in a parallel position so your stance is fully supported.
- Remember to breathe from your stomach at all times so you do not put any tension in your face and neck.
- When you stand, try not to slouch, and use your stomach muscles to pull you up rather than taking all of the strain in your legs and back.
- When you walk, breathe deeply and feel as if a thread is attached to the top of your head. Allow the thread to pull you upwards so you are walking tall and your neck and spine are straight. Keep your stomach and buttocks tucked in.

## Exercise 16: Chiropractic and Reflexology Adjustments

- If you are having any neck or back pain or finding that your posture is being inhibited, see a chiropractor. Chiropractors do not just correct spinal abnormalities, but they also remove blockages in the spine which result in interference with the nervous system. Since the nervous system controls all functions of the body, including the immune system, chiropractic care can have a positive effect.

- I recommend the Activator Method chiropractic technique which is a gentle, low-force approach to chiropractic care using an instrument rather than manual adjustment. Try to find an Advance Proficiency Activator chiropractor in your area.
- You can also release pressure points on your feet by simply massaging your own feet. The reflexology points for the neck are at the base of the big toe and the points for your spine run down the inside of your foot. Your middle back reflexology point is located on the top of the foot. Massage your feet every night while you are watching television or ask your partner to give you a foot massage. This will help to release any neck or back pain. The massage may feel painful at first until you have released the blockages. Keep pummeling away, and you will soon find relief.

**Exercise 17: Supplements**

Taking a high grade multivitamin and mineral supplement will help you build muscle mass. For strong bones take a calcium supplement and maintain your Vitamin D levels. You can also add the following minerals and amino acids to your diet to strengthen and tone your body.

- **Boron** is a mineral that is naturally found in fruits such as apples, prunes, pears, and grapes. Vegetables like carrots, leafy greens, nuts, and grains are also rich sources of boron. Boron supplements help build strong bones and muscles.
- **Iron** is an important mineral that helps with blood circulation and transportation of oxygen to the body. Iron also works with myoglobin, a protein that helps supply oxygen to the different muscles. Foods rich in iron include leafy green vegetables, spinach, beans, and cereals.
- **Creatine** is a supplement that helps improve muscle strength and muscle growth. Creatine works by providing energy to the muscles in

order for them need to work properly. Food sources such as fish and meat products contain creatine.

- **Glutamine** is an amino acid famous for contributing to quality muscles. Glutamine is generally available in the form of instant soluble powder from most health food stores.

### Exercise 18: Healing Your Posture with Crystals

- For personal power, place hematite or abalone shell on your solar plexus.
- For lack of grounding, place black agate, hematite, or tiger's eye on your root chakra.
- To connect to your spirituality, place tourmaline, ruby, jade, or aquamarine on your crown chakra.
- If you suffer from backache, place a long piece of selenite under your mattress or lie on your front and place it on your spine. Carry sapphire, turquoise, or if the back pain is coming from muscle damage, carry jasper, aventurine, or topaz.
- For general aches, hold magnetite or rose quartz to affected areas.
- For cramps in legs, wear, carry, or hold chrysocolla.
- To help with the flexibility of your joints, wear, carry, or hold azurite or malachite.
- Carry aventurine for sore muscles; for posture wear amethyst.

# 7

# True Beauty Comes from the Heart

*Beauty is not in the face;*
*beauty is a light in the heart.*
**Khalil Gibran**

You are nearing the end of your spiritual program. By reading this book you have absorbed vast amounts of spiritual information and have learned an array of practical exercises to help you spiritually, mentally, emotionally, and physically transform. You are moving closer to a place of perfected love to help you heal your body and to slow your aging process. But for you to have a true inner and outer beauty glow that radiates out to the world, we first need to define the meaning of true beauty. I define it as being your authentic self at all times. Beauty is finding the real you. If you live and love as your authentic self from your open heart, you will reflect your pure soul. Beauty is not about physical perfection but about learning to open your heart and to love yourself. You are beautiful when you are a confident, loving person who knows who you are and who lives and loves as God guides you, no matter the consequences or the reactions of the outside world. True beauty comes from the heart and soul, not from a bottle, plastic surgery, or a pill.

I know that many of you reading this would also agree. So why, if we understand and agree with the quote by Khalil Gibran, do we still not really believe we are beautiful deep down inside? Why do we continue to look outside ourselves for validation and stare at our face in the mirror every day instead of focusing on the love in our heart and the emotions in our soul?

The heart is a reflection of the soul condition; it reveals the truth of who you are. Just consider: when someone asks you to identify yourself, where do you always point? Do you point at your head? Do you point at your feet? No, you point at your heart. You instinctively know that your heart and your soul (which is also connected in the chest) are the real you.

How many times have you met someone who is externally gorgeous, but her cutting sarcasm and hardened heart repels you as soon as she opens her mouth? Or have you met a handsome male model, but your heart sinks when you realize he is emotionally disconnected? Then you see a fifty-year-old woman who is vibrant and confident and all eyes go to her, or you feel attracted to a silver-haired man because he respects himself and everyone else in the room. You realize that age does not matter; it is all about energy and the way people love. You feel people's hearts and their souls, and they either attract or repel you, no matter what they look like on the outside.

The truth is that most people are afraid to open their hearts every day because it makes them feel vulnerable. As you learned in previous chapters, they live from their controlling minds and egos rather than from their open, loving souls. They perpetuate the reactionary, intellectually competitive masculine era in the world rather than embrace the new feminine era of reconciliation, intuition, cooperation, and feelings. They become scared to love and long for love because they have been so let down in the past or have never received it. They are scared because of their previous experiences with love, and they wait for someone to love them before they can love in return. Even then, some people panic when they receive love. Their hearts constrict with fear because the love entering their souls triggers the release of their stored emotional pain. Instead of letting love enter to heal them and allowing the pain to pour out of their system, they sabotage their relationships, shut down their hearts, and turn their backs on love. But the soul is the center or the truth of who we are, and the sacred, intuitive heart is the place we must return to if we want to be happy, healthy, and living our best life.

## THE POWER OF THE SACRED HEART

But how much do you really know about your heart apart from the fact that it beats and pumps blood around your body? This complex organ and correlating heart chakra energy point in your spirit body is not just a vital organ to keep you breathing; it is a powerful navigator and healing center that guides you through life, rejuvenates you, and heals every cell in your body. Because the heart chakra also acts as the master chakra for the lungs, the act of breathing serves to activate the thymus. The thymus is a ductless gland associated with the functioning of the heart chakra. It is one of the earliest glands to develop in the fetus while in the womb. It also has much to do with telepathy. It is available to anyone that knows where it is and how to open it. It is located in the middle of the chest about three inches above the nipples, to the right of the heart, which is why it is often referred to as the high heart. It sits between the heart and throat chakras, an area where intent originates, connecting the emotions of divine love, compassion, truth, and forgiveness with the area where language originates—hence the meaning "speak from the heart."

The word "thymus" is derived from the Greek *thymos*. In modern terms it can be translated to denote a life force, soul, and feeling or sensibility. It is known as the seat or the abode of the soul. I believe it is the joining point for the soul, i.e. where the soul connects to the etheric and physical body. When you put pressure on the thymus, it is painful to touch. When you touch the thymus, all the grief that you have stored in you comes pouring out. Just as the womb stores deeper emotions, the thymus or thymic chakra is our main grief center.

A good way to balance the physical body is to work with the breath and the energy of both the heart chakra and the thymus gland. When you breathe deeply, as in meditation, and gently tap on your thymus, the heart energy flows smoothly to produce that sense of calm and relaxation. And when you breathe while focusing on the heart chakra, you will flood your system with the light energy of unconditional love.

When you have an openly and unconditionally loving, nonjudgmental heart which loves you and others deeply, the energy of that love radiates throughout your body, creating an energetic cellular reaction which heals the body and changes how you look and feel. It is the love that flows from your heart and soul which lights up your face and radiates your beauty out into the world. It connects you to the fountain of youth.

Ancient Egyptians celebrated the heart rather than the brain. Egyptians believed the heart was the main intelligence center—a sacred, intuitive emotional beacon that healed with its power and light. They noticed that when a person felt sad, excited, or angry, it was the heartbeat that changed, and this was why the Egyptians thought that the heart, not the brain, was the seat of wisdom and knowledge. The importance of the heart was reflected in Egyptian burial practices. The Egyptians were very concerned with the survival of the heart. It was the only major organ that was left inside the corpse. They made efforts to remove the brain and did not even bother to preserve it, unlike the other major organs that they removed and preserved. For additional protection, a separate heart in the form of a heart scarab was also provided at the burial in case something happened to the deceased's heart.

This knowledge about the heart is becoming known by more than Egyptologists, many doctors, scientists, and spiritual teachers refer to the heart as the second brain. They say it has a complex nervous system that is in constant communication with the brain.

The popular mainstream doctor Dr. Christiane Northrop claims that "the heart's electromagnetic field is sixty times larger than the brain's."[2] Scientists at the Institute of HeartMath claim in their research publication that the heart's ECG measurements are also about sixty times more powerful than the brain's EEG measurements and the magnetic current generated by our thoughts is five thousand times weaker than the magnetic qualities of the heart.[3] This is why people fail when they use spiritual intellectualisms and mental affirmations or try to "think" abundance

---

[2]Christiane Northrop, *Women's Bodies, Women's Wisdom* (New York: Bantam Dell, 2006), 649.

[3]Institute of HeartMath Research Staff, *Science of the Heart: Exploring the Role of the Heart in Human Performance-Publication No. 01-001* (Boulder Creek, CA: Institute of HeartMath, 2001).

into their lives or manifest happiness through meditation. As I have repeatedly stressed throughout the book, the Law of Attraction is the desire that comes from your feelings, not your thoughts. You cannot heal your soul or change your Law of Attraction just by changing your thinking; you can only fully heal by releasing the negative feelings which create the thoughts so that the electromagnetic charge of the emotion is permanently released from your body.

The power of the heart cannot be denied. It is highly intelligent and a powerful carrier of information. It can be trusted more than the mind and can help you determine what is good and what is bad. It will release a chemical to let your brain know that you are making a good decision. The circuitry of the heart is so sophisticated that it also has a memory and can sense and feel. It sends the brain extensive emotional and intuitive signals. The Institute of HeartMath claims not only to have proven scientifically that the heart's electromagnetic field is the most powerful rhythmic field produced by the human body, but also states that it extends out in all directions into the space around us. The electromagnetic field envelops every cell of the body and connects you to every other sentient being on the planet. Human beings electromagnetically bond through love. That is why it is so important that you keep your heart open at all times if you want to stay safe, informed, healthy, and connected.

Anyone can receive knowledge through the heart; he or she just needs to learn how to access it. So how do you learn to receive information? It begins with dropping down from your mind and focusing your attention on your heart to activate its electromagnetic potential. It also begins by the understanding that the heart is always contracting and expanding. When the heart expands and opens fully, then its intuitive, loving power can heal, create miracles, and connect you deeply to everything and everyone around you. But when you shut the heart down because of your fear and emotional injuries, you block love from flowing in and out, which stops you from receiving vital information and sending clear messages to the brain.

The blockage of the heart means that you not only become disconnected from yourself, but it also isolates you from others. As you block the heart and put up an invisible wall, a membrane starts to grow across the heart chakra, blocking its light further so the healing rays of your heart cannot work. This membrane acts as a protective shield, and as it grows, your electromagnetic field and sensory ability become greatly reduced. When you break through your emotional blocks, your soul and your thymus expand, and the heart chakra membrane breaks. When your heart expands and opens again, you will often feel chest pain in your sternum. You may also feel heart fibrillations as both the thymus (high heart) opens and your heart chakra membrane tears apart. Some people say it feels like indigestion or a mild heart attack. But it is not an ailment; it is just the heart bursting open to its full capacity and returning to its natural state so that it can heal you and radiate love out to the world.

Opening your heart to love is not going to cause a heart attack. The thing that is going to stop your heart beating is your fear and emotional blockages. The shutting down of your heart hardens your heart's arteries. The thymus is a gland that produces many of those disease–fighting soldiers—the white blood cells that come to your defense against many types of infections. If it is not functioning properly and the thymus chakra is blocked, it can be implicated in a wide variety of disorders, especially ones that involve the immune system. A broken heart can literally mean just that. Blocked grief causes heart disease and heart attacks as well as such diseases as lung cancer. We learned in Chapter 5, emotions of disappointment and loss can cause acidity and disease by changing the body's cells.

Living with an open heart is a very freeing experience. It also helps to create miracles because the intuitive powers of your heart and your telepathic abilities of your thymus develop, which heightens your senses. You can feel, sense, and connect to everything around you even if you are far away from someone or something. This extra sensory ability can be a good thing, but it can also be difficult at first because up to this point your blocked heart has been numbing you from everyone and everything around you. When your heart is fully open, the lack of feeling stops. You will be aware of the feelings of others as well as your own—the baby crying down the street, a couple in love, an animal suffering, or the hunger pains of the starving millions who live in India. Once your heart is open, you are fully activated and aware of all the joy and suffering in the world, including your own and other people's. This is the true meaning of being alive.

"But how," I hear you ask, "can we stay open and love fully without fear? How do we remove the protective shield around our heart when the world is a cruel, competitive place and people hurt us by their actions?" To make ourselves vulnerable again after all the difficult experiences of the past can be a frightening thought. But to live without an open heart and never to risk loving fully means your life will be cut short both in time and in meaningful experiences.

Spiritual masters have an excess of energy and live lengthy lives because they do not waste any of their energy on hating anyone or being afraid. Their hearts are opened fully, and they love unconditionally at all times—no matter how anyone else behaves. They believe that love is the greatest weapon of all, and because they understand God's laws and have fully awakened to who they are, they know who the person standing in front of them really is, too.

When you are in a place of total, unconditional love for yourself and others, you will never be tired; your energy will remain abundant and your heart will function properly, healing everything in its sight. As an opening occurs within you, your body will vibrate at a different frequency and rejuvenate your cells. Your energy will also affect others. You will electromagnetically charge other people without them being aware of it. This is how the global heart and sense of interconnection grows. But unfortunately, so many are preoccupied with their own selves and their physical vehicle that they forget about their hearts; they become emotionally disconnected and have no clue how to love themselves or another human being.

As you have learned throughout this book, this shutting down of the heart began when we were children. When you were young, you loved everyone openly; you did not feel "self" conscious or separate your "self" from others because you were free from emotional injuries. You lived from your heart and your soul, and you were free from all self-criticism.

But as you grew older and people started criticizing, restricting your free will, and telling you what to do, your damaged soul condition started to activate your negative thoughts and feelings, tricking you into believing that you were different from other people and not good enough. You felt you must protect and defend yourself from others in case they criticized and hurt you again. That is when your heart shut down and became entirely blocked.

Unfortunately, as you have learned in this book, your powerful emotional injuries do a lot of damage. They drive your whole life by dividing and destroying. The hatred and fear in your heart leaches energy from you and harms those around you. Your fear blocks you from giving and receiving while the energy you put into attacking, avoiding, or ignoring someone depletes you. Your anger consumes the healthy, loving pure energy that runs through your cells, and your bitterness shuts down your heart, causing blockages, ill heath, and an untimely death.

The only emotion that can overcome all your mental, emotional, spiritual, and physical destruction as well as the destruction of others is love. This is the pure love that emanates from your heart and soul to yourself and others. It is God's Divine Love that flows into you and transforms your soul. Darkness cannot affect love, because it cannot grab hold of it. It is on a denser plane of vibration, and it is not even interested in love. That is why when we stay in a place of love, we are always protected. But love cannot enter you if you have a barrier around your heart and you shut out the light that wants to enter you. That is why an integral part of your daily practice should be to love, cherish, and open your heart, no matter the circumstances so that its light protects you and performs at optimum capacity.

## WHAT IS LOVE?

Each soul has the personal capacity to develop its love for all things in its environment. The biggest problem that stops most people from loving themselves, their partners, and other human beings is that they do not understand what love is and is not.

They have learned that love is painful, self-sacrificing, demanding, exhausting, and conditional. They have learned to believe that they are unlovable and worthless and that they should sacrifice themselves for the benefit of other people. They have also learned to harm themselves emotionally, physically, and spiritually. These disharmonious, error-filled beliefs about love became ingrained because of the unloving beliefs and action of others in their environment.

That is why God's guidance system tries to help you align with the truth about love. If you are in harmony with God's laws of love, you will love yourself unconditionally; you will not self-sacrifice, hurt yourself, or treat yourself unlovingly in order to love others. You will always be emotionally honest and nurture yourself. You will never physically abuse yourself. You will not respond to others' demands or expectations for your love. You will understand that your love is a gift. If you feel complete love for yourself, you will never need anyone else to love you in order for you to be happy. You will have no expectations either. You will not feel hurt if others do not do, say, or feel what you expect them to.

This is why your heart opening begins by learning God's laws of Natural and Divine Love. Whenever you cannot treat yourself or other people the way that God treats you, you know that you have emotional errors or false beliefs about love to release. Whenever you are in conflict with another, you have both forgotten how God loves. You are stuck in emotional injuries and need to release the false beliefs and desires about love that are not in accordance with God's laws. If you can understand how God loves and understand what love is and what love is not, then you can begin to manifest healthier relationships and live a happier life.

Putting the laws of love into practice into your own life starts with a question. Every interaction with your partner, family member, or another person should start with the question: "What does love do?" But because we are often injured in our understanding of love, perhaps a wiser question would be: "What does God's Love do?" Our emotional injuries often cause us to have a warped view of love and usually manifest as a lack of self-love, selfishness, or unloving actions towards others. When we ask: "What would God's Love do?", we can try to see our partner and ourselves as God sees us. God believes that our feelings and our partner's feelings are equal in importance. Therefore, when you interact with your partner, you both should ask questions about how you can each love as God loves. For the sake of the following example, I am considering my partner as a male. You should imagine the words to refer to your specific situation. You would first ask yourself:

- What would my love for myself motivate me to do for myself?
- What would my love for my partner motivate me to do for him?
- What do I feel my partner's love for himself motivates him to do for himself?
- What do I feel my partner's love for me motivates him to do for me?

Your partner can ask the same question from his own perspective:

- What would my love for myself motivate me to do for myself?
- What would my love for my partner motivate me to do for her?
- What do I feel my partner's love for herself motivates her to do for herself?
- What do I feel my partner's love for me motivates her to do for me?

Using God as an example of how to exemplify the true meaning of love may sound like a very obvious thing to do, but with pressures from family and friends, a dose of low self–esteem from your father, and love injuries from your mother, exemplifying God's Love can be incredibly hard to follow in life. If you can stay in truth and ask yourself the above–mentioned questions every time you interact with another, especially your partner or your children, and then process the emotions that come with the answers, you will then be well on the way to trans–forming your relationships.

Let us learn more about love and continue to answer the questions: "What would God's Love do?" and "What would God's Love not do?"

## 1. LOVE IS UNCONDITIONAL

God loves unconditionally and gifts you love whether you love God or not. When you are in harmony with God's laws of Natural Love, you will love people even if they do not love you in return. When you truly love, you can love people even if they disagree with you. Most people are in disharmony with God's laws of Natural Love because they give a service or a gift only when others react positively. They do not give their love as a gift—they love only if they get something in return. Their love is conditional. Do you still love someone in your life even if that person has turned his or her back on you? I would imagine that if your answer were no; you have probably contracted your heart and put a protective shield around it. You probably feel that this person does not love you so you will not love him or her or that this person has hurt you so you will not love him or her back. That's why 99 percent of people on the planet do not love in the unconditional way that God loves because they do not understand the true meaning of love. God never stops loving you even if you do not love in return. This is how you need to love yourself and others if you want to unconditionally love as God loves.

## 2. Love Is not Self-Sacrificing

Even though it is important to love others unconditionally, you will see that when you love in the right way, you will never allow others to treat you unlovingly. If they are unloving to you, then you remove yourself from the interaction. You should also immediately address issues when other people treat you badly. You have probably been taught that if you are a loving person, then you should sacrifice yourself and your desires for the benefit of other people. But to truly love as God loves, you do not sacrifice your own happiness or your desires for another; otherwise you would be unloving towards yourself. For example, if your partner is an alcoholic or a drug addict and continues with the addiction that results in the destruction of your own life, then you need to ask: "What would love do?" If you loved as God loves, then you would not allow another person to cause chaos in your life, and if that person loved you, he or she would not continue to drink too much, take drugs, or damage you. Love is not about self-sacrificing for another human being or harming yourself. That is a distorted viewpoint of what "love" is. Ultimately it will be your own examples of personal boundaries, emotional honesty, and self-love that will help the people around you learn how to love themselves.

## 3. Love Does Not Have Expectations

True love holds no expectations. God desires but does not demand your love. When we demand love or try to manipulate or guilt-trip people into loving us, we are being unloving. If individuals choose to gift you love or do something nice, they are activating their own free will to love you. But they also have that same free will to choose not to do something for you or not to love you. If you respond in a negative way towards them after they choose to follow their free will and say no to you, then you are the one in the wrong because you are violating their free will. Love is a gift, not an expectation or a manipulation.

This also applies to how others love you. If you are to follow God's laws about love, you will not believe that others can, through their angry outbursts, demand love from you and try to control, manipulate, or guilt-trip you into doing what they want. You will never change your loving behavior even when others get angry with you.

## 4. Love Is Emotional Honesty

As you have learned in previous chapters, love means being emotionally honest at all times, no matter the consequences. Too often we are taught that others' emotions are more important than our own and that the only way we can receive love is by earning it. We have also been taught to believe that we are responsible for other people's pain. Most importantly, we lie to others about our true feelings so that we do not cause them further pain. If you are honest about your true feelings to yourself and others, no matter the consequences, you will always be in harmony with God's Love. When you lie about how you really feel, you are actually being unloving to yourself and the other person. Truth telling sets you free and helps your soul condition. Tell the truth at all times and process the emotions that well up in you when you do. This also allows the other person to process his or her own emotions.

## 5. Love Honors Everyone's Free Will

If people really love you as God loves you, they will always honor and support your free will. It is true also that when you love people as God loves, you always honor their free will whether or not you agree with their decisions. You will support and encourage them to experience their emotions. They are allowed to do, feel, or be whatever they want even if they go completely against Divine Truth. If you do not honor others' free will, they will feel they are being controlled by you which will propel them into rebellion and they will harm themselves further. They will feel suppressed and sense that they cannot have their own emotional experience. They may also feel obliged to please you— just as children do with their parents. They will often repress their own feelings or desires, which will harm their soul condition and make them feel frustrated and angry.

If you do not honor others' free will, you, too, will feel annoyed or frustrated because they are not doing or feeling what you want them to or are not agreeing with you. You will also feel that you are better than they are and that they do not understand. All of these behaviors are unloving. Your unloving, controlling behaviors have been caused by emotional injuries. You have been taught as a child that people prove their love to you if they do as you want—and vice versa. Your need for control is because you want to avoid your own emotions about feeling unloved.

## 6. Love Is Nonjudgmental

Judgment in any form is unloving. In fact, judgment can be as harmful as the worst of crimes because judgment can kill. Judging others can drive them to their death. Judging yourself can also lead to ill health and your subsequent death. If you judge others, it simply means that you still judge something inside of yourself. If you judge yourself, you are perpetuating your parent's judgment of you when you were young. When you love yourself completely as God loves you and you have cleared your emotional injuries, you will no longer judge yourself. When you love yourself unconditionally, you will not judge other people either, no matter what they have done. God never judges, no matter the mistake, the crime, or the circumstance.

## 7. Love Encourages Passions and Desires

When you love yourself, you will always follow your passions and desires as long as they are in harmony with God's Truth and Love. You will never suppress your desire because of feelings of obligations placed on you by others. If you emanate love to others, you will assist them to develop their passions and desires if they are in harmony with God's laws. If others' passions and desires are in error, you will not assist them, but you will not try either to stop their free will or judge them, even if this means letting them go from your life. If you do not help someone and it is in your power to do so, you will feel a penalty on your soul. This refusal to help others is usually because you have a deep feeling of selfishness or envy and you feel sad that you have not fulfilled your own passions and desires in your life. But at the same time you will also feel a penalty on your soul if you help them do something that harms them.

## 8. Love Addresses the Cause But Not the Effect

What I sow, I will reap. When you love yourself and others as God loves you, you do not try to change your life or another person's life by changing the effects. You focus instead on addressing the cause. If you treat only the effects, the cause will continue. Everything that happens has a soul-based cause within you or another. If you take away only the effect of a person's emotions or actions, you will feel tired, disappointed, and unfulfilled because you are not addressing the cause. You will probably find that others take advantage of your assistance and do not thank you because you are assisting them to stay in their error. You should never intervene to mitigate the effects unless the people are willing to address the cause. It is actually unloving to deal just with the effects because they will never fully heal. They have to desire change. Your desire to help usually stems from an addiction to feeling important and a denial of your own causal pain.

## 9. LOVE FOLLOWS THE LAW OF ATTRACTION

When you do not follow your own Law of Attraction, you stop your soul growth and stay in self-denial. You then do not love yourself as God loves you. You unlovingly punish others rather than feel the deeper causal emotions they trigger in you. When others treat you unlovingly, deal with the emotions in yourself rather than retaliate. You should not hate, blame, seek vengeance, dismiss, or desire to punish others, no matter how they treated you. Likewise, if you do not show people their Law of Attraction, you allow them to remain a victim in their own lives. You enable them to not take responsibility for their own creations so they can never clear the deeper emotional pain within themselves that created the Law of Attraction. When you love others as God loves, you encourage them to see that everything that happens is the result of their Law of Attraction.

## LEARNING TO LOVE YOURSELF AND OTHERS

Now that you understand how God loves and what love would do and would not do, you can begin to unblock your heart and love yourself. Your love for yourself will radiate through your body and rejuvenate your cells. Once you fully love yourself, as God loves, you will be capable of extending unconditional love to others.

This process may take time because most people do not love themselves in any shape or form. They are full of self-loathing and completely out of harmony with God's Love. This stems not only from their childhood injuries but also because of false societal prejudices, fears, and belief systems inflicted against them, such as the public shaming and condemnation of homosexuals or the fear and prejudice projected onto black men.

These issues appear different from the outside, but they are connected and lead to the same place. The unloving, false beliefs perpetuated against the gay community have driven many to their deaths and have caused millions to self-abuse and loathe themselves. Likewise, the fear and racism projected onto black men as they walk down the street have left many feeling hopeless, unloved, and still segregated. Many black males have unfairly fallen foul of the justice system. Like the homosexual soul, many have turned their inner pain to a life of selling or taking drugs. They, too, want to numb the misery they feel about a world that judges and condemns them. As they disappear out of sight behind barbed wire fences and prison cells, they, too, are given a clear societal message over and over again that they are worthless and they are not wanted.

Just as oppressed women around the world need to collectively rise up and become equal through overcoming their fears, releasing their grief, and loving themselves, so we must encourage young black men and homosexuals to do the same. We must support the black male so he can heal his angry, ostracized heart, and we must strive to help him remove the physical and spiritual chains that have shackled his mind, body, and soul since the dark days of slavery. We also need to support and encourage all homosexual soul halves on the journey back to finding their true soul mate and a place of perfected love.

Both communities have the potential to become new leaders in the new feminine era—powerful carriers of the Divine Masculine and Feminine if they can learn to love and accept themselves fully. We must hold a sacred, loving space for all the so-called societal "misfits" as they take their rightful places at life's table, release their grief, forgive the fear and bigotry, heal their wounds, and learn how to love themselves deeply. We should also forgive and hold a space for those who have persecuted others for their differences. They, too, will need to heal and release their fear and grief. Many of their judgmental or abusive behaviors have been due to multigenerational emotional injuries as well as false societal and religious belief systems.

As I discussed in Chapter 2, awakening to the fact that the beliefs you have followed all of your life may be wrong in God's eyes can feel terribly painful. It can rock the foundations of people's lives and turn their whole world upside down. But from that place of Divine Truth and new beginnings, they, too, can heal and start to live life in a healthier and more peaceful way, respecting and embracing all parts of themselves and other people while living a life built on a more solid and truthful foundation that is aligned with both the feminine and masculine aspects of God.

## THE BEAUTY MYTH

The media has also perpetuated an intense sense of self-loathing in our society by propagating a myth about perfection. Since you were born, you have been bombarded by images in the media that have made you feel imperfect, unlovable, and unworthy. You have been told that you will be loved and desired or be of some value only if you purchase material things. You have been told you are lovable only if you are young, thin, and wearing the designer product the advertiser is selling. Men have been told that they are not successful and women will not desire them if they do not drive the right car, earn the right amount of money, or carry the latest technological gadget. There is no mention or revering of a male in the media if he heals his own soul and learns how to love properly. Consumerism is kept alive by playing on people's fears and emotional injuries. Advertisements terrorize us with images that suggest we will be lonely, unloved, and worthless unless we look like the young celebrity or airbrushed model on the magazine cover. This beauty myth controls people—especially women.

The beauty stereotypes have set up a system of competition and envy. They have created divisions and kept women from being empowered and collectively uniting. When we allow the system to control us, we will always remain small and unworthy. We will never be a true leader, and our soul will never fully expand. We will look and behave as someone else—usually the latest fad celebrity or model. Remember, true beauty comes from your authentic self so if you are living as somebody else, wearing someone else's nose, or facial expression, then your inner beauty will not be revealed or shine as brightly.

In God's eyes, we are all perfect. Our imperfections are perfection. They give us our individual frequency, specific quality, and vibrational note. Each freckle, crook of our nose, or kink of our hair reveals our unique soul, here to play a special role. As the years go by, the wisdom we accumulate from the ups and down of our individual lives should be celebrated because it expands our souls even further. God knows that it is our imperfections and mistakes that help us grow and return to our pure self. The Buddhists compare humans to lotus flowers that are growing in mud. The mud or manure is needed to feed the flower and help it blossom fully into a beautiful flower. You are not defined by your mistakes but how you overcome them. If you had not gone through the problems in your life or made mistakes, you would never have matured into the person you are today. Every pearl needs a grain of sand in the oyster shell to cause irritation so it can gradually grow and be transformed into a precious jewel.

When you reject the beauty myth, embrace your imperfections, your age, and your shadow self while following the non–dualistic philosophy discussed in Chapter 2, you stop the "either . . . or," the "better than," and the "different to" dialogue that is constantly running through your head and separating you from other people. You understand that no one is perfect, including you. There would be no day without night, light without dark, and good without evil. From this place of acceptance and wholeness, you will stop judging yourself and others so harshly. Remember, judgment in any form is unloving and goes against God's harmonious laws of love.

This dualistic, judgmental belief system is also being perpetuated in society by the paparazzi and tabloid press whose daily life is dedicated to either revering people or condemning them. Their salacious and often cruel articles that publicly crucify anyone who looks and acts less than perfect are powerful examples of the shadow self. These unloving, judgmental behaviors reveal that the journalists and photographers working for the magazine are themselves full of self-loathing. They are condemning others because they still judge something inside of themselves. Those who buy and read the magazines are also judging because of a lack of self-love. Their desire for gossip comes from trying to avoid their own life issues and deeper painful emotions. What they do not realize is that as they devour the tabloid news stories and magazines, the celebrities' lives they read about are symbolic of their own. They are watching heightened scenarios and scandals play out to highlight the issues in their own lives. As both journalist and reader continue to revere or condemn something outside of them, they are avoiding the clearing of their own soul. This denies them the experience of discovering their own inner celebrity and standing in their own spotlight. Next time you buy a newspaper or gossip magazine, you need to ask yourself the question: "What am I avoiding inside of *me* that is making me more interested in you?"

As for the subjects on the cover, all their feelings of unworthiness which have been inside of them since childhood are being triggered through their Law of Attraction so their souls can heal. Once the emotional injury has been healed, then they will no longer create a negative Law of Attraction in the form of a tabloid story. Much of their desire for fame has come from the same early childhood injury. Their desire for public approval and recognition led to their successes, but the unworthy feeling and emotional injury that drove them to seek fame in the first place has never been fully addressed. This is why the celebrity has attracted in a negative attack by the press.

Society has put a price tag on everything. Money has become more important than love, competition more important than compassion, image more important than emotional truth and authenticity. The media needs to ask itself the question: "'Is my story healing or harming?" In fact, all humans need to ask if their words and actions heal or hurt.

Yes, indeed, we all need a dose of self-love and a guidance system that can show us how to open our hearts again, heal our souls, and return to a place of nonjudgmental and unconditional love. As I spoke about in Chapter 2, no matter our current beliefs about God or religion, we all need a guiding light, a goal, or a target—something more perfected than we are to lead us down the correct path to happiness and love. When we treat others with a lack of care, compassion, and respect, we then know that there is something inside of us that needs healing.

God is inclusive, not exclusive. God loves all people no matter who they are. God looks beyond the superficial invisible barriers that separate humans. God is colorblind, loves variety, and has no labels, especially not designer ones. God loves all people no matter what they look like, how much money they have, or how they worship. To God the outside is not who we are. God knows that the real you is on the inside.

When you love as God loves, you will celebrate uniqueness and start to experience peace and interconnectedness with everyone and everything. You will not judge someone by what he or she looks like on the surface. You will transcend differences in religion, political beliefs, gender, age, social standing, culture, and race. You will never separate gay from straight, rich from poor, black from white, and women from men. Everybody is created in the image of God so if we judge others or turn our backs, we judge God and turn our backs on the Creator.

If you use God as an example, you will step outside of your comfort zone and your inner circle. You will release your sweeping generalizations. You will not judge the outside but will discover who someone is on the inside. Speak to someone who is not from your country, who does not follow your religion, who is not the same skin type, sexual orientation, or social standing. You may be surprised at what you find. If you set your prejudices aside, you will receive God's blessings, and your life will be full of new knowledge and experiences.

Do not judge people's individual journeys either. Try to find compassion for people's destructive behavior or the circumstances of their lives. You do not know their stories: Were they abandoned by their parents? Did they grow up poor or in a wealthy, abusive family? You do not have to excuse their behavior, but you can find compassion for them as you discover the truth about why they behave in a certain way. As you learn about the story of their lives, count your blessings that you did not have to suffer the same fate.

Only God sees the bigger picture and understands the reason why certain things are happening. Everyone is being prepared for a greater destination, just as you. When people face disaster and their lives are stripped bare, they are being given the opportunity to connect to their pure soul, rise up out of the ashes, like a phoenix, and soar. Lives go up in flames to burn off impurities and emotional injuries. As the saying goes: "The harder we fall, the greater we rise." Every crucifixion or personal tsunami is an opportunity to experience a spiritually positive change of life.

God would want us to pay particular attention to those most vulnerable. We should open our hearts to children, the sick, the elderly, the poor, and those in trouble. God did not create an abundant planet so a few could own everything while others have nothing. Every human being in the world should have shelter, clothing, food, water, and healthcare. If that is not happening, then the system is showing it is sick and broken. The winner-takes-all approach is out of harmony with God's Truth and Love. If you have accumulated great wealth in your lifetime, then help your neighbor. Remember, we are alive so we can love; we are not here to live for the love of money. You cannot take your material riches with you when you die, but you can gain great spiritual riches through developing compassion. The love in your heart will help you continue a prosperous life on the Other Side.

We should also open our hearts to animals. Animals are not here for our entertainment, to gamble on, or to provide us with a fashion product. They, too, are God's children, and like our own children, they are our most vulnerable of citizens and the greatest of our teachers. The presence of an unconditionally loving animal in a person's life can greatly heal his or her body, mind, and soul. An animal is always emotionally present and loving to its caregiver. No matter what is going on around them, dogs will always wag their tails and want you to throw a ball. Animals are meant to be treated with respect at all times. Any person keeping a bird or an amphibian in a small cage in their home is being unloving, anyone doping horses and forcing them to race, selling puppies in a profit-making mill, poaching wild animals for their skins or tusks, coercing elephants to stand on their hind legs and juggle in a circus, using monkeys for commercials, movies, or tourist's photos, anyone forcing dogs or cockerels to fight in a back street so they can win a bet and, most especially, anyone taunting and killing an unassuming bull with a sharp sword in a Spanish arena is being unloving. Any audience member watching, cheering, or supporting these violent and degrading acts will also incur a penalty on his or her soul because they, too, are being unloving. An evolved person does not harm animals. When we harm an animal or treat them with anything less than complete respect, we then are showing the world that we are not conscious; we are full of self-loathing. We do not love or respect ourselves either. Gandhi stated that: "The greatness of a nation and its moral progress can be judged by the way its animals are treated." When we lose respect for animal life, we lose respect for human life as well.

When you love as God loves, you let your heart expand, and you go beyond the traditions and bigotry that have been passed down through your family line. You know you are God's child, and you have a world full of brothers and sisters, both animal and human, whose blood is red, just like yours. Pure light is made up of every color of the rainbow so open your heart fully and fill it with the light and love of every corner of the world.

## LEARNING TO FORGIVE

The art of opening your heart and loving begins with the practice of forgiveness. Forgiveness is the key to learning to love yourself and others. It helps you open your heart fully so your body can rejuvenate and heal. Every wise man or woman understands the strength it takes to forgive another. Gandhi knew that forgiveness is "the attribute of the strong and that the weak can never forgive." He was also passionate about the importance of not retaliating and causing others harm just because they had harmed you. Consider his famous quote: "An eye for an eye makes the whole world blind." It sums up how no one wins if we retaliate rather than forgive.

Forgiveness is not easy to ask for, and it is even harder to give. It is even more difficult to forgive when someone has not even asked for forgiveness. That is why forgiveness is a process, but a process we must all go through if we are to be set free from negative emotions.

Because God gave everyone free will, we do not have to forgive if we do not want to, but if you do not forgive someone, then you will be hurting yourself. Holding onto emotions such as anger or bitterness inside of your system can cause a lot of damage both to yourself and others. Ultimately, a refusal to forgive turns into resentment and resentment is an energy-sapping emotion that always hurts the sender more than the recipient. If you do not forgive, the anger in your heart and soul will damage your body. These harmful emotions will lower your frequency and accelerate your aging. They will also affect the environment around you. As you project your suppressed emotions, you can potentially make other people ill.

There are four steps to forgiveness. If you follow these steps listed below, you can free yourself from resentment and any wrongdoing—either by yourself or another. There is no reason to refuse to forgive in any situation. God forgives instantly so try to follow God's example.

# 1. Forgiveness Is an Emotional Process
## Forgiving Yourself

Forgiveness can take time; it is an emotional process that needs to be honored and done properly. If you have harmed another, then you must feel the depth of your own emotions about the event. If you have hurt another, then you need to explore the causal reasons why you harmed him or her. You can then ask for forgiveness for your actions. Perhaps you have cheated on your spouse or have been abusive with your language or actions. You need to process emotionally rather than punish yourself. Self-punishment is unloving and a waste of time. If you do not forgive yourself and uncover the root cause of your actions, then you will not heal. If you do not heal, you will probably do the same thing again. If you keep punishing yourself and hold onto unloving emotions such as guilt or shame, you can cause yourself a lot of emotional, spiritual, and physical damage.

Forgiveness is also not about allowing the other people to punish you. If they are focused on punishing you and being angry, then they, too, are avoiding their causal emotions. Just take responsibility and do not avoid how you feel about those actions, thoughts, words, or deeds that are not in harmony with love.

If you have hurt others, you will still feel the emotion generated by your action, but you will also feel the forgiveness of God. God freely forgives you, so you should be able freely to forgive yourself. If you can free yourself from guilt and shame, you will not treat others as if they are better than you. When you judge yourself and do not forgive yourself, you prevent yourself from forgiving others because you will be judging them, too.

## Forgiving Others

How do we forgive people when they have hurt us so badly? What if they have killed a loved one, stolen our life savings, physically or mentally abused us, or perhaps, betrayed us and left us with a broken heart? How can we possibly forgive those who have caused us so much pain and ruined our life? If you refuse to forgive, you are trying to avoid feeling your own emotions. You should rather be willing to work through the causal emotions until they are released from your soul.

Forgiveness is a process of clearing all our emotions of hatred, blame, anger, and bitterness. It is also a process of grieving for what you might have done differently—for the innocence, trust, and free will you feel you have lost. Most of the time, people are more angry with themselves for letting someone hurt them than they are with the perpetrator. So the first step to forgiveness is to forgive you for not loving yourself enough. It was your lack of self-love and your emotional injury in your soul that allowed something harmful to happen in the first place. Once you forgive yourself, you can move on to forgive the people who have hurt you.

Forgiveness is about understanding the part you played in the circumstances of your life. In a situation where people deliberately meant to harm you because of their emotional injuries and when you truly understand the Law of Attraction, you will accept that you, too, were partly responsible and had something present in your soul condition that attracted the event. Everything in your soul that is in harmony with Divine Truth and Love protects you from harm in the external environment. If the contents of your soul had been completely harmonious, you would have been fully protected.

If a crime was committed against you, then there was obviously an emotional charge radiating from your soul, attracting in another negatively charged person or event. Maybe your self-esteem was low when you were abused by your husband or you felt unworthy when you had all of your money stolen or you did not trust men and were fearful when you were followed home late at night. We are all partly responsible for any negative event in our lives. If you can be honest and answer hard questions about how you felt when you were a victim at the time you were harmed, then you can start to forgive. If you can accept that you were partly responsible for what happened, you will not feel like a victim and will be able to forgive those who have sinned against you.

You can accelerate your process of forgiveness by praying to God to help you release all the causes of why you cannot forgive and what caused your Law of Attraction in the first place. This will help you return you to a place of love. A lack of forgiveness prevents you from becoming at one with God because you will never be free of all the negative emotions you hold onto because you are in denial.

However, as I have said, just because you take part responsibility for an event does not mean that you should punish or blame yourself. Self-blame, guilt, or shame is a waste of your precious energy. Your emotional injuries were probably caused by your childhood so were not your fault. Move beyond self-punishment and find the emotion that caused your Law of Attraction.

## 2. Forgiveness Is Emotional Forgetfulness

Many people think they have forgiven someone, but the well-known saying "I forgive, but I'll never forget" really means a person has not yet fully forgiven. If you have not forgotten, you have not really forgiven.

When you have truly forgiven and released the negatives emotions around your past experience, you will not remember what happened in the first place; you will have no residual emotional charge or signature in your soul against the event or person. Forgiveness could be described as emotional forgetfulness. Use this theory to help guide you to feel whether you have completely forgiven someone or not.

Forgiveness is not an intellectual exercise; emotional forgetfulness comes from deep within the soul. So if you are still rejecting a person, harboring feelings of anger and resentment, or even remembering what someone did to you in the past, you need to process your negative emotions because you are yet to truly forgive and that is hurting your body.

Until you have learned to forgive, you will never be free from suffering. If you can understand and face the fact that you would rather punish someone than feel the painful emotions about what happened to you, you will feel trapped. But when you have forgiven, you will be free of all these painful emotions.

## 3. Forgiveness Is Following the Law of Attraction

Your Law of Attraction is your messenger of truth. Your Law of Attraction will reveal to you when you have truly forgiven. If you have forgiven, you will not avoid or fear meeting those that have hurt you, unless they choose to repeat their harmful actions. You will feel no more anger or resentment towards them.

## 4. Forgiveness Is Releasing All False Beliefs

Another reason that we find it hard to forgive is because many of us have been taught that God is a punishing God. We believe that God is a wrathful entity who thinks we are sinners and destined for hell. When we clear societal mistruths about God, we can then start to forgive. If you believe that you are an eternal sinner, it will be hard to forgive yourself and others who have sinned against you. You will continue to punish them just as you feel that God punishes you. You will feel that you are a bad person who is guilty and can never be good enough.

As I discussed in Chapter 6, this false perception of God comes partly from false religious belief systems and partly from how our parents have treated or continue to treat us. Remember, our relationship with our parents is reflected in our relationship with God. If your parents always put you down or were angry with you, then you will also believe that God thinks you are bad and wants to punish you. If you can create boundaries and disallow any harmful or negative treatment of you or projected blame by others, then you can learn the real truth about love and forgiveness while healing your relationship with yourself and with God.

## Learning to Show Mercy

Many people struggle with forgiving someone who has committed a harmful action because they feel the other person does not feel sorry for what they have done: they have never apologized or made amends. If you are struggling to forgive someone, remember, you can free yourself from carrying harmful emotions in your body and soul by instantly forgiving them, just as God instantly forgives. But that does not mean you have to take them back into your life or show them mercy if they have not shown remorse. It is actually more loving not to show people mercy until they are sorry because otherwise they will never learn their lesson and heal. They will harm themselves or someone else again.

The Law of Mercy also applies to us. If we have let go of the emotions that caused us to harm another, we are instantly forgiven, and as long as we repent, we should follow the Law of Mercy and be merciful on ourselves. Repentance is the key to letting go of a situation and experiencing the freedom of forgiveness. The problem is that because of our feelings of unworthiness, we continue to punish ourselves for our past errors. We are often not as merciful towards ourselves as we are to others.

Then there are those who are quite the opposite; they show themselves mercy before they have even taken responsibility for their own harmful actions. They want to avoid any emotional pain or responsibility. But if they do not own up to their own mistakes and feel remorse for the harm they have caused, the emotional penalty in their soul will never go away.

Remember that when our actions are in error, our soul attracts the penalty as soon as we break the law. The consequences of sin are always emotional, and penalties are stored in the soul emotionally. The sin or error occurs whether or not we are conscious of it; although if we are conscious of the error, then the penalty on the soul is greater. If we are sensitive, we will feel the penalty in our soul immediately.

Many people load the word "sin" with guilty undertones although the true meaning of "sin" translated from Aramaic is "missing the mark" or "missing the mark of perfected love." It simply means we need to correct an error within ourselves because our soul emotions are disharmonious with God's Love. This is caused by childhood emotional errors that have damaged the contents of the soul. It is these errors that entered the soul which create all love injuries. It is the love injuries that create all sin. Another reason sin happens is because error often enters the soul disguised as truth because our emotional injuries create a belief that something is loving even when it is not loving from God's perspective. If you harm people or people hurt you, then they are not living in a consciously loving state and are failing to live by God's laws. It does not mean that you or they are to be damned for all eternity. If you can process your emotional errors, you can stop feeling as if you are in hell.

Centuries ago archers used to shout out the word "sin" when they fired a bow and arrow. The word was used to declare that someone had missed the target so they needed to take another shot. It was not cloaked in heavy guilt or judgment. This is also true of the word "evil." The word "evil" means "unripe" in Aramaic. It was used to describe an unripe fruit or someone who was not fully matured or developed spiritually. People were described as being ripe or unripe rather than being good and bad. An unripe person was seen as not yet being evolved or conscious, not ready, and not in rhythm with life. They are unloving because they have not awoken to the truth of who they are. They have not cleared their negative emotional injuries and addictions.

When people have cleared their negative emotional injuries and have healed their love injuries, they have awoken to the whole truth of who they are and they do not harm another. Only the unloved and unenlightened have fear and hatred in their hearts. All actions stem either from the emotion of love or the emotions of fear or shame and the like. If people have harmed you, they are fearful of feeling their real causal emotions; they are lashing out at someone else and projecting their own dark shadow-self onto you. Happy people, who love themselves completely, share only their light.

This is why we have to give people access to higher knowledge and compassionately encourage them to keep taking another shot until they are on target; as Maya Angelou stated, "When you know better, you do better." If we lock up criminals for life, throw away the key, and leave them rotting in jail, then we are being unforgiving and therefore unloving in God's eyes, especially if they are remorseful. Further still, if we mercilessly inflict the death penalty on a murderer, then we, too, are committing a felony. Any person who orders the killing of others is a murderer in God's eyes—whether they are an army general ordering his soldiers to kill in wartime or a judge ordering an execution of a prisoner on death row. God gave us the free will to kill but the killing of others, no matter what they have done, is a spiritual crime. People involved in killing or ordering others to kill will inflict a heavy emotional penalty on their souls. This penalty will seriously degrade their soul condition. The karma will have to be dealt with by the person in this life or when he or she has reached the Other Side. As Gandhi said, "we all become blind if we retaliate." God never added an addendum starting with "but" or "unless" to any of the universal laws. Remember, the truth will set you free from suffering as long as you bring your personal truth and your personal beliefs in harmony with God's Truth which is the absolute truth and not your version of it. We, too, will have lost our way if we stop following the laws of God and God's law is not to kill under any circumstances. If you find this concept hard to accept, let's consider the case of self-defense. If you have cleared your emotions and fears about being harmed or dying, then your Law of Attraction will probably not attract in such a harmful event that would trigger the need for self-defense. It is our fear-based feelings and actions that cause killings so it is important to choose love over fear in these instances.

Besides, the Law of Compensation takes care of anyone who is disharmonious and who is violating God's laws of love. The Law of Karma inflicts an emotional penalty on any erring soul until there is remorse. The higher spiritual law automatically starts a process to bring a person back to a place that is harmonious with love. The current penal system does nothing to contribute to the healing of others or to the mending of their hardened hearts. It does not heal any of God's "unripe" children or help them to take responsibility for their crimes. It is merely keeping prisoners locked up in pits of hell without any hope or tools for rehabilitation. This means that if or when prisoners are released, they often go back and commit the same crime again due to unresolved emotions of anger and self-loathing.

Because the conditions of most prisons are so inhumane, violent, and abusive, the prisoners inside also becomes victims or even greater abusers. This means that they never truly own up to what they have done or make amends for the harm they have caused. They remain angry and never face the emotional reason of why they did their harmful actions in the first place. They are given food, prison clothes, and housing but never have to take responsibility for their own lives. It would be better to give them spiritual teachings to help them clear their emotional wounds and multigenerational injuries, tools to grow their own food, materials to make their own clothes and build their own houses so they could start to learn how to love and nurture themselves. When people learn the acts of self–love, they learn how to respect and love others. Once a prisoner is healed and is no longer a risk to the community, he or she can then return to society and contribute in a positive way.

Those who have been victims of a crime also fail to heal. Victim and perpetrator are kept apart by lawyers so there is no restorative justice, no truth talking, and no taking of responsibility by either party for their Law of Attraction. On top of that there is no clearing of emotional injuries, no healing or redemption, and no opportunity to forgive. The victim's soul condition also becomes degraded by the unresolved negative emotions he or she never gets the opportunity to process.

God would never create a system that does not give people the opportunity to return to a place of peace, love, and harmony. Neither would God lock people in the darkness of their pasts and stop their souls from expanding into the light. God's laws are always trying to move people back to living harmoniously in the present moment of their lives.

Prisoners who are given the opportunity to rehabilitate themselves can transform themselves into profoundly wise and knowledgeable spiritual men and women because they have been given the time to reflect and be still. Their incarceration brought them closer to their Creator and the truth of their own souls. A healing has occurred. Their newly healed selves should be embraced and used for a higher purpose. They are also God's children, our brothers and sisters; their transformational stories serve as powerful messages of healing for all of us. It is only our own fear that keeps us locked in a state of unforgiveness. As we bind the hands and shackle the feet of men and women and refuse to unchain our own hearts, we send out a clear sign that we do not love or forgive ourselves either.

All people can correct an emotional error and make amends at any time in their lives, including you. All people can release negative emotions, let love enter their hearts, and ripen with the correct spiritual knowledge and assistance. There is always a possibility for liberation, redemption, forgiveness, and healing, no matter the crime. When you love as God loves, you can instantly forgive and show mercy to yourself and others because you understand the root cause of harmful actions. You can transform your angry, vengeful, unforgiving heart into one of love, forgiveness, and compassion.

## LEARNING TO HAVE GRATITUDE

You can keep your heart open and in a space of love if you accept where you are today and return to a place of gratitude. When you make peace with your life, accepting your current circumstances and your Law of Attraction, you can work through all of the causal emotions that are degrading your body and soul. If you do not accept where you are and punish yourself about the past or feel frustrated that you are not where you want to be in the future, you will not be present to your real emotions. If you are not emotionally present, then you cannot keep your soul pure because you will be avoiding the how and why you got to where you are today.

When you feel gratitude, your heart opens because you see that everything which has happened to you in your adult life is perfect. You will start to feel gratitude for your past experiences as you come to understand that you would not know joy if you had not known sadness. You would not know what success feels like if you had never failed. You will also realize that those who have hurt you have been your greatest teachers. These people were your own Law of Attraction. They showed you the truth of what needed to be healed in your soul. You can feel gratitude for the fact that these people helped you face your greatest fears and your darkest emotions, and they triggered your emotional addictions and injuries so the addictions and injuries could come to the surface for you to clear.

You were never a victim! Your soul condition brought people and events into your life to help you realign with God's Love. Learn to be grateful for your mistakes, however hard they may have been. Remember, you are here on earth so your soul can experience individualization, self-awareness, and growth towards God. The past events and mistakes have been wonderful life lessons to help you evolve. Taking responsibility in this way and finding acceptance and gratitude for all your interactions will help you keep your heart open and accelerate your healing process so you can return to a place of perfected love much sooner.

## How to Build a Healthy Heart

You can physically help to strengthen your heart by exercising and breathing properly. Conscious breath work is one of the best ways to improve rib cage mobility and open the heart space. The muscles tighten around the heart as a result of defensive breath patterns. As you learned in Chapter 3, any time people feel threatened and feel the need to guard or defend themselves or avoid their painful emotions, they usually hold their breath or breathe in shallow, erratic patterns. These shallow breaths not only affect the muscles round the heart but also produce tension in the upper abdomen which restricts normal movement of the diaphragm. These restrictions affect the amount of oxygen flowing through your body. Keep practicing the breath work exercises from the previous chapters to deepen your breathing and relax the muscles around your heart. You can also gently stretch the thoracic soft tissues with specific yoga poses, such as a backbend practice. The backbend can really help to open the heart area, both physically and energetically. It will help you learn to become vulnerable and open to love. There are more examples of yoga exercises at the end of this chapter.

Healthy eating is also going to be an essential part of keeping your physical heart functioning properly. Eating and exercising in the right way will support your spiritual practice as you remove the emotional blocks from your heart. Remember, taking care of your inner and outer temple is an act of self-love. Follow the nutritional and exercise suggestions in the previous chapters. There are also dietary and exercise suggestions at the end of this chapter that are specifically designed to strengthen, open, and support your heart. Make sure you walk every day, eat a low cholesterol and low sodium diet packed full of antioxidant fruits, vegetables (especially spinach), garlic, ginger, herbs, fish, whole grains, and essential fatty acids. Garlic especially helps regulate the body's blood pressure. Whether you have problems with low or high blood pressure, garlic can help equalize it.

Many doctors recommend that heart patients take a CoQ10 supplement. When heart tissue cells are 75 percent deficient in CoQ10, the heart ceases to function. CoQ10 is a prescription heart medication in Japan. It plays a vital role in the treatment and prevention of heart disease and improves the heart's ability to pump more blood. In the past few years, there has also been an increased interest in the role that magnesium plays in preventing and managing conditions like high blood pressure and cardiovascular disease. Take a daily magnesium supplement or eat fish or nuts regularly to maintain magnesium levels and a healthy heart.

## CONCLUSION

Now that you have learned about forgiveness and the power of your heart, you are aware of your greatest health and beauty weapons. Love cures all things, transforms all things, and heals all things. Inner and outer health and beauty do not come from material possessions, plastic surgery, or a person's status in life. They come from loving yourself, your soul mate, other people, and God. If you stay in a place of love, everything in your mind, body, and soul will transform. Your life will change for the better, and your relationships will get healthier and stronger, too.

You have reached the end of this powerful program. You are equipped with spiritual tools, higher knowledge, and practical exercises to purify, rejuvenate, and transform your body. You have all the tools you need to become a spiritual master. You are now a self-healing and self-replenishing divine being. If you remain dedicated to this program, you will release all of your emotional, mental, and physical toxins and shift to a place of perfected love. From this state of light and Godliness, your body will operate from the highest frequencies—the fountain of youth.

As you progress with self-mastery, you will acquire the desire to be more disciplined, and it is this discipline that will reconnect you to your health and beauty. The rejuvenation of the mind, body, and soul must become part of your everyday schedule. You have to carve out quality time for yourself to ensure the tools you have been given have a lasting effect. This is all part of the new life for the new you. You deserve to dedicate yourself to a life of self-love.

It is now time to share your metamorphosis. It is time to find the courage to live your light. Go share your heart and radiate your beauty out to the world. Be a living example of heaven on earth. You have found true beauty because you have found your authentic self. Remember that there is no set weight or age that defines beauty. God made only one of you, so go be an original—your own original shape, size, and energy field. Live from your pure soul, and your body will naturally return to the perfect vessel that God intended for you.

Hopefully you now realize that you are a sovereign unto yourself—a superhuman with extraordinary powers who can transform all things through the power of your soul. Do not play small or apologize for your greatness. Let others experience the powerful frequency of your knowledge and love, so that they, too, may discover their true beauty, connect with their soul, and remember who they are.

No matter your age, no matter your past, your soul is aching to expand and live to its full potential. Let your authentic self fly free, no matter what anyone else thinks or feels about you. Live from your unique childlike spirit, breathe deeply, eat healthily, and exercise daily, feel instead of think, connect deeply to your heart instead of your intellectual mind, stay emotionally humble, release destructive ancestral blueprints, heal your multigenerational, intergender wounds and childhood injuries, reunite with your soul mate, balance your yin/yang schedule, surrender and simplify your life, let nature and children guide you, follow your Law of Attraction, always speak the truth, forgive your enemies, love unconditionally as God loves, and rediscover your passions and desires. You are not alone on your journey. Seek God and develop your faith. You will always be rewarded.

Most importantly, remember that it is not your age that defines you but the contents of your soul. Live from your pure soul, and you will stay forever youthful. Reside at the highest level of perfected light and love, and you will live a life of eternal grace and beauty as you experience the best years of your life. As George Eliot once said, "It's never too late to be who you might have been." Be yourself and you will fulfill all of your lifelong dreams.

## • *Exercises for the Sacred Heart* •

### Exercise 1: Connecting with Your Heart

- Hold your hand on your heart chakra in the center of your chest. Focus your energy and attention on your heart. Feel your energy drop down from your head to your heart. Feel the different sensations in your heart. Start thinking with your heart instead of your head. Imagine your heart is leading you as you walk down the street. Imagine your eyes are actually in your heart, leading you wherever you go. Keep practicing this exercise until you feel that your heart is beginning to lead rather than your head.

### Exercise 2: Learn to Love Yourself

- Write a list of all of your good points, your best traits, and everything that you love about yourself. Are you funny, happy, unconditionally loving, compassionate, or helpful? Absorb all of those positive traits that are unique to you. Keep releasing any negative childhood causal emotions inside of you that make you feel unlovable or unworthy.

### Exercise 3: Learn to Soften Your Heart

- Find a picture of someone you love. Notice how your heart feels. Now find a picture of someone you hate with whom you have an ongoing dispute or whom you are ignoring. Do you feel your heart contract and harden. Keep looking at the picture and feel all of the emotions that well up inside of you. Remember, it takes two to create a relationship and two to break it. Take responsibility for your part in the breakdown. Remember that the other person was your Law of Attraction. You attracted them in from your damaged soul. Feel the emotions inside you until you have released them. Allow the fear, anger, and hatred to spill out while the truth and love come in. Feel your heart soften and open once again.

**Exercise 4: Learn to Open Your Heart**

- If you are a Democrat or Liberal or a Conservative or Republican, get a picture of a former or current political leader and look at the picture until your anger subsides and you feel peaceful with your adversary. Try to find someone who has opposite political views to yours and practice speaking with him or her.
- Make a mental note of your feelings when you are dialoguing; then go home and process all the negative and positive feelings inside yourself. Better still go to a Republican/Conservative or Democratic/Liberal meeting. Breathe deeply and stay there until you have cleared your anger, division, and hatred.
- Interact with anyone who is not of your faith, not from your culture, or not from your country. Note what you both have in common, even if you approach things in a different way. Do you both love your family and friends? Are you both trying to make a living and give your children the best education? Do you both believe in God? Visit a church, synagogue, or mosque that is different from your own.
- Find a person at a party with whom you would not normally speak, perhaps someone who dresses differently from you. Have a conversation with him or her. Take note of how you feel during your discussion. Did you feel your heart open more as you were speaking or did it shut down and get angry or frustrated. Go home and work through these emotions.
- These exercises may take some time; you may have a lot of biases, anger, judgment, frustration, and sadness to release, but once this exercise is completed, you will be able to walk on the planet with a heart open to all people, no matter your differences.

**Exercise 5: Activating the Thymus Gland (Higher Heart)**

- To open your thymus, look at your chest area just above the heart and take several gentle, focused breaths directed at that space. Tap the thymus. It may feel sore at first. You will notice that you are breathing differently than you were a few moments before. Release your stored grief.

**Exercise 6: Finding Forgiveness**

- Acknowledge the injury or the hurt within yourself caused by an event or a person. Experience the painful emotions of the hurt. Think about your Law of Attraction and how you were feeling at the time you were harmed.
- Grieve about the event until you no longer feel any emotional attachment to it. Release the emotion that caused the attraction in the first place.
- Pray to God for help to forgive and to remove the cause within you that prevents you from forgiving.
- Visit the places, locations, or people that caused the event to see if you still have a negative, emotional reaction. The people you have forgiven will often feel differently towards you and change in their actions.
- When you have found forgiveness in your heart and soul, show mercy to the other person once he or she has taken full responsibility, learned the lesson, and repented.
- Write to prisoners. Share this book with them. Show them that they are not alone and someone believes in their redemption.

**Exercise 7: Finding Gratitude**

- Write a list of all the things that you are grateful for. Allow yourself to experience the love you feel for all whom you love in your life. Feel your heart expand as you do this exercise.
- Write a list of all the people who have harmed you in your life. Process emotions about them until you experience gratitude for the lessons and how they helped you become aware of the injuries in your soul through your Law of Attraction.

**Exercise 8: A Healthy Heart**

- Exercise regularly and get plenty of fresh air. Walking is especially good for the heart.
- Become vegetarian or cut down on meat, especially fatty red meats and processed meats such as sausage, salami, and hot dogs, etc. Choose

lean meats such as chicken or turkey and remove the skin. Meat fat can cause high cholesterol, and it adds excessive weight.

- Eat fish, instead of meat, at least twice a week
- Increase fiber and whole grains
- Reduce sodium—too much salt raises blood pressure. Use herbs and spices instead.
- Spinach has high potassium and low sodium content. This composition of minerals is very beneficial for high blood pressure patients. Spinach proteins also reduce cholesterol and other fat deposits in the blood vessels. Folate present in spinach contributes in reducing hypertension and relaxes blood vessels, maintaining proper blood flow. A pigment named lutein found in spinach has been shown to reduce the occurrence of heart attacks, strokes, and atherosclerosis (the hardening of arteries.)
- Eat plenty of garlic and ginger to lower cholesterol.
- Cut down on dairy foods. Use skimmed or low fat milk and low fat cottage cheese, sour cream, or mozzarella. Substitute egg whites for eggs yolks.
- Use liquid vegetable oils such as olive, sunflower, or coconut instead of butter and lard.
- Drink green tea. It is effective in lowering cholesterol levels and inhibiting the abnormal formation of blood clots.
- Take fish oil; it contributes in reducing cholesterol. The risks of coronary heart disease are also cut down by the fiber content in flaxseed meal.
- Take a CoQ10 and Vitamin D supplements to prevent heart disease.
- Take olive leaf extract and Manuka honey to boost the immune system and add protective qualities for the heart and circulatory system.
- Take a magnesium supplement to lower blood pressure.
- Epsom salts helps prevent heart disease by lowering blood pressure, protecting the elasticity of arteries, and preventing blood clots. Bathe in Epsom salts regularly.

**Exercise 9: Heart-Opening Yoga Poses**

There are a number of well-known heart-opening yoga poses that effectively open the chest and abdomen. Practice breathing in each position for two to three minutes a few times a week if not every day. If you do these exercises every day, you will be rewarded with deep relaxation and an opened heart space. Do not push yourself too hard but rather gently, breathe and stretch.

- Place a folded blanket, small pillow, or a yoga roll lengthwise under your spine. Bend your knees and place the soles of your feet together at the midpoint of your body, about six inches from your main torso. Support your head so it is slightly higher than your chest. Breathe deeply. This position gently expands the front rib cage, upper abdomen, and heart area.
- To expand and loosen the chest area even further, you can do a series of simple twists. Lie on your right side with your knees pulled up toward your chest so you create a 90-degree angle at the hips. As you inhale, open your left arm behind you while turning your head to the left. Repeat this exercise to the other side; lie on your left side with your knees pulled up. As you inhale, open your right arm behind you while turning your head to the right.
- **The Bridge Pose** not only opens your chest but increases flexibility and suppleness while strengthening the lower back and abdominal muscles. Lie down and place your feet on the floor so they are parallel to each other. Place you hands under your buttocks and gently raise your lower back and tail toward the ceiling. Lower your back to the floor. Repeat this exercise a few times and then continue to raise your lower back, lifting the spine until your entire back is arched upwards. Push firmly with your feet and raise your chest. Keep your knees straight and close together. Clasp your hands under your back and push against the floor. Breathe deeply for five seconds, then release. As an alternative, you can keep your hands down by the sides to push yourself up, or you can lift your arms back over your head to rest on the floor behind you.
- **The Chest Fly** is also beneficial to people with heart chakra issues. Sit with your legs crossed. Raise your arms to your sides with your palms facing up. Rotate your arms forward, stopping just before your palms meet; then rotate them back, spreading your chest open. Repeat this slowly for five minutes.
- **The Camel's Pose** is a backbend that stretches the front of the body, especially the chest, abdomen, and quadriceps. It helps to unblock the

heart and improve spinal flexibility. Begin by sitting up onto your knees. Draw your hands up the side of your body and reach your hands back one at a time to grasp your heels. Move your hips forward so that they are positioned over your knees. Let your head come back and allow your mouth and throat to open. Do not tense. Breathe deeply.

- **The Upward-Facing Dog Pose** opens the front of the body. Lie on your stomach; place your hands on the ground beneath your shoulders. Gently push up extending the arms as far as is comfortable. Try not to lock the elbows or strain the lower back. Lift the chin to arch the head back and open the heart. Try not to tighten the jaw line, the buttocks, or the muscles in the lower back. Breathe slowly and deeply to maximize the heart-opening effects of the pose.

### Exercise 10: Healing Your Heart with Crystals

- To heal a broken heart, hold, wear, or carry chrysocolla or elbaite. Place a piece on your heart chakra.
- For a closed heart, hold, wear or carry eudialyte or green kyanite. It opens the heart to love.
- For an unforgiving heart place green dioptase on your thymus chakra.

# Bibliography

*Angelic Revelations of Divine Truth—Volumes 1 and 2.* Recorded by James E. Padgett. Santa Clarita, CA: FCDT Publishing, 1989.

*Book of Truths.* Recorded by James E. Padgett and compiled by Joseph Babinsky. Prescott, AZ: Gentle River Publishing, 2010.

Gleason, Marion N., Robert E. Gosselin, and Harold C. Hodge. *Clinical Toxicology of Commercial Products: Acute Poisoning (Home & Farm).* Baltimore: The Williams & Wilkins Co., 1957.

Institute of HeartMath Research Staff. *Science of the Heart: Exploring the Role of the Heart in Human Performance–Publication No. 01-001.* Boulder Creek, CA: Institute of HeartMath, 2001.

McCarthy, Jenny and Jerry Kartzinel. *Healing and Preventing Autism.* New York: Plume Publishing, 2010.

Northrop, Christiane. *Women's Bodies, Women's Wisdom.* New York: Bantam Dell, 2006.

Permutt, Philip. *The Crystal Healer.* London, England: Cico Books, 2007.

Stone, Joshua David. *The Complete Ascension Manual.* Flagstaff, AZ: Light Technology Publishing, 1994.

# About the Author

Victoria Holt is an internationally renowned spiritual counselor, writer, journalist, and producer who is well-known for her down-to-earth approach to the healing of the mind, body and soul of individuals and mass audiences through one-on-one counseling and global multimedia. She has spent twenty years training in spiritual traditions of all faiths and has worked with world-renowned spiritual leaders, corporations, celebrities, and everyday people who are looking to heal their lives.

She has written for national newspapers in England and has appeared on television and radio, both in England and America. In 2004 Victoria wrote and directed the documentary *A Walk of Wisdom*. The film had its world premiere at the Santa Barbara Film Festival in January 2005.

Prior to her spiritual work, Victoria trained as an actress and dancer at the London Studio Center. She gained a Bachelor Degree in Dance at Middlesex University, England. She has trained in screenwriting and film production and as an on-air host at the ITV studios in London. Victoria also worked for five years at J. Walter Thompson Advertising and KLP Marketing but gave up the commercial world to sell something she believes in—spiritual living.

Victoria has developed shows for Disney and the SyFy networks partnering with Golden Globe and Emmy winners. She is currently working with a team of producers to launch a television show based on this book, *Spiritual Facelift*.

Victoria would be interested in reading your comments about the book. You may contact her at www.spiritmediainc.com.

# 4TH DIMENSION PRESS

## An Imprint of A.R.E. Press

4th Dimension Press is an imprint of A.R.E. Press, the publishing division of Edgar Cayce's Association for Research and Enlightenment (A.R.E.).

We publish books, DVDs, and CDs in the fields of intuition, psychic abilities, ancient mysteries, philosophy, comparative religious studies, personal and spiritual development, and holistic health.

For more information, or to receive a catalog, contact us by mail, phone, or online at:

**4th Dimension Press**
215 67th Street
Virginia Beach, VA 23451-2061
800-333-4499

## 4THDIMENSIONPRESS.COM

# EDGAR CAYCE'S A.R.E.

### What Is A.R.E.?

The Association for Research and Enlightenment, Inc., (A.R.E.®) was founded in 1931 to research and make available information on psychic development, dreams, holistic health, meditation, and life after death. As an open-membership research organization, the A.R.E. continues to study and publish such information, to initiate research, and to promote conferences, distance learning, and regional events. Edgar Cayce, the most documented psychic of our time, was the moving force in the establishment of A.R.E.

### Who Was Edgar Cayce?

Edgar Cayce (1877–1945) was born on a farm near Hopkinsville, Ky. He was an average individual in most respects. Yet, throughout his life, he manifested one of the most remarkable psychic talents of all time. As a young man, he found that he was able to enter into a self-induced trance state, which enabled him to place his mind in contact with an unlimited source of information. While asleep, he could answer questions or give accurate discourses on any topic. These discourses, more than 14,000 in number, were transcribed as he spoke and are called "readings."

Given the name and location of an individual anywhere in the world, he could correctly describe a person's condition and outline a regimen of treatment. The consistent accuracy of his diagnoses and the effectiveness of the treatments he prescribed made him a medical phenomenon, and he came to be called the "father of holistic medicine."

Eventually, the scope of Cayce's readings expanded to include such subjects as world religions, philosophy, psychology, parapsychology, dreams, history, the missing years of Jesus, ancient civilizations, soul growth, psychic development, prophecy, and reincarnation.

### A.R.E. Membership

People from all walks of life have discovered meaningful and life-transforming insights through membership in A.R.E. To learn more about Edgar Cayce's A.R.E. and how membership in the A.R.E. can enhance your life, visit our Web site at EdgarCayce.org, or call us toll-free at 800-333-4499.

**Edgar Cayce's A.R.E.**
**215 67th Street**
**Virginia Beach, VA 23451-2061**

## EDGARCAYCE.ORG